Creating Health

Books by Deepak Chopra, M.D.

Creating Health
How to Wake Up the Body's Intelligence

Return of the Rishi
A Doctor's Story of Spiritual Transformation
and Ayurvedic Healing

Perfect Health
The Complete Mind/Body Guide

Quantum Healing
Exploring the Frontiers of Mind/Body Medicine

Deepak Chopra, M.D.

Creating Health

How to Wake Up
the Body's Intelligence

Houghton Mifflin Company   Boston

To
MAHARISHI MAHESH YOGI,
whose extraordinary insight into the nature
of intelligence restructured my reality

Copyright © 1987 by Deepak Chopra
Introduction to the 1991 edition copyright
© 1991 by Deepak Chopra, M.D.

For information about permission to reproduce selections
from this book, write to Permissions, Houghton Mifflin
Company, 2 Park Street, Boston, Massachusetts 02108.

Library of Congress Cataloging-in-Publication Data

Chopra, Deepak.
Creating health.

1. Medicine and psychology.   2. Mind and body.
3. Transcendental Meditation.   4. Health.   I. Title.
[DNLM: 1. Health Promotion—methods—popular works.
2. Preventive Medicine—popular works.   3. Psychosomatic
Medicine—popular works.   WM 90 C549c]
R726.5.C53   1987   613   86-20019
ISBN 0-395-42953-6
ISBN 0-395-57421-8 (pbk.)

Printed in the United States of America

BP 10 9 8 7 6 5 4 3 2 1

Portions of this book were published by
Vantage Press in 1985.

Grateful acknowledgment is made to Harper & Row,
Publishers, Inc., for permission to quote excerpts from
The Upanishads, translated by Alistair Shearer and
Peter Russell, copyright 1978 by Peter Russell and
Alistair Shearer.

Contents

Introduction

Creating Health was written in one long burst of excitement. I dashed away from Boston to a cabin in Vermont and started writing furiously. My brain was fired by a revelation, my spirits soared as high as the clouds over the Green Mountains. I had the key! I was going to reveal a secret beyond price.

My inspiration came from a simple phrase: the mind-body connection. At first these words sounded rather colorless, but in them I could hear the sound of walls crashing down. Mind and body had long been separated by a very old, very thick wall. The mind was a ghost, the body a machine. They occupied totally separate domains, as far as medicine was concerned. I had never known anyone to see, touch, measure, or weigh any connection between them. The most prestigious medical journals ridiculed the notion that sickness and health might depend upon anything as shadowy as the patient's mind.

But now that would change. The mind-body connection was real, and here was the proof — a flood of "messenger molecules," barely understood before the late seventies, that course through the bloodstream, transforming our most intimate thoughts, emotions, beliefs, prejudices, wishes, dreams, and fears into physical reality. Mind turns into matter, not at the high point of a magic act, but as the ordinary business of the body's fifty trillion cells. You cannot experience the faintest mood without your heart cells sharing it, and at the same time your lungs, kidneys, stomach, and intestines. These organs participate in your mental life as fully as your brain does.

Everything the mind can conceive is projected onto a 3-D screen that we call the body. We do not in fact have a body and a mind but a bodymind, one seamless web of intelligence that expresses every flicker of intuition, every shift in the configuration of an amino acid, every vibration of an electron. Our intelligence cannot be a ghost in a machine because the machine is itself intelligent, and that means it isn't a machine at all. I think that this is the crowning discovery of twentieth-century medicine.

I wrote *Creating Health* to inspire people who may not care about norepinephrine or serotonin until they are shown the revelation that lies behind the dry chemical names. When they truly see the body, they understand that it is completely fluid. It flows like a river and changes as quick as lightning. The old model of the body as a sculpture frozen in time and space must be discarded, because that model keeps us in the grips of disease, aging, and ignorance. As the later parts of the book show, the mind-body connection can take us past all limitations. It is like a thread that begins in our DNA, crosses the threshold of the brain, and leads onto the portico of the universe.

Such knowledge is too huge to be straitjacketed by medical science — it must be lived to be appreciated. In that sense, *Creating Health* is unabashedly a manual for living. It seemed to me that people should be given a taste of what it is like to be totally free of boundaries. Reality is not a given; it is a possibility that we shape and control. The problem is that our society has not taught us to be skilled reality-makers. Instead, we are taught to respect our status as reality's prisoners. An Indian disciple once asked his master, "Why do I feel so bottled up inside?" The master answered, "Because everyone feels that way." I realized that many readers would be experiencing exactly this kind of frustration; in response, I have laid out the knowledge of a higher reality, based on the assumption that human awareness was created to achieve total freedom.

I didn't write with any one person in mind, but I hope these chapters will make a difference to Anna, a Boston woman in her mid-fifties who came to see me last week with a highly emotional story. Several years ago she discovered some small, discolored bumps on her right cheek. The fear of cancer flashed through her mind, but her dermatologist assured her that all she had were harmless sebaceous cysts. He scraped them, gave the affected site a few injections of cortisone, and pronounced her cured. Anna went home, expecting to feel relieved, but she could not shake off the recurring suspicion that she might have cancer nonetheless.

She consulted a second dermatologist and insisted that a biopsy be taken. He reluctantly complied and was not surprised when the biopsy came back negative. Anna was now diagnosed with a "non-specific skin inflammation" that was definitely not malignant. However, driven by some unnamed intuition, she insisted upon a second biopsy, which again came back negative. Now her doctor gave her a stern lecture about not letting fear get the better of her, and Anna went away.

Three days later she received an embarrassed phone call. The lab reports had somehow gotten mixed up, and her doctor was sorry to inform her that she did indeed have a rare type of cancer known as an atypical melanoma. She underwent immediate surgery, followed by a course of radiation, at the end of which she was again pronounced cured.

To everyone's intense irritation, she could not accept this verdict. She still felt that something was very wrong, and soon a routine chest x-ray disclosed that the melanoma had moved into her lungs. This time there was no treatment that could completely eradicate the malignancy, but after another course of radiation, Anna was told that her disease had responded well. She was now considered to be in remission.

Throughout these ups and downs Anna's emotions were constantly tossed between hope and despair. Her dread of doctors became pronounced, and when she developed a chronic chest cough a year later, which coincided with a death in her immediate family, she had little tolerance for medical intervention. She permitted an x-ray under one strict condition: "Whatever you find, don't tell me the results."

The radiologist agreed, but a few hours later he returned to her hospital room. "Look," he said, "I've got good news for you. Don't you at least want to hear it?"

"If it's good news," Anna murmured doubtfully, "I suppose there's no harm in knowing what it is." Whereupon she was told that there was nothing abnormal about her x-rays. Her lungs appeared to be free of disease.

"I don't believe it," she replied adamantly. She demanded that her x-rays be forwarded to the prestigious cancer clinic that was treating her case. Her oconologist examined the films and called her in puzzlement. "What do they mean, nothing abnormal?" he said. "The same malignant nodules are present as before. Your old and new x-rays are practically identical."

And so her case stands today, winding its way through a tragi-comedy of medical errors and blind alleys. The only reliable element in the whole sad story has been Anna's feeling, her intuitive sense of self, and that is the very thing each doctor consistently ignored. Now Anna feels extremely distraught and angry. The most terrible result of all Anna's tests is not that she has cancer, but that her chief defense against disease — her ability to feel comfortable and secure — was systematically stripped from her.

So what can I do for Anna now? I will try to give her back what she has lost. We need to turn the mind-body connection into the channel of life, which is after all our home. The same deep sense of self that warned Anna about her disease should also be able to cure it — at least that will be our working assumption. Since it is not an easy assumption for some people to accept, laying it out in detail helps. With that in mind, I offer *Creating Health* to Anna and to all the other people who want to make their own reality, free from fear and intent upon freedom.

I

Health and Disease

1

How to Be Perfectly Healthy and Feel Ever Youthful

HEALTH IS OUR NATURAL STATE. The World Health Organization has defined it as something more than the absence of disease or infirmity — health is the state of perfect physical, mental, and social well-being. To this may be added spiritual well-being, a state in which a person feels at every moment of living a joy and zest for life, a sense of fulfillment, and an awareness of harmony with the universe around him. It is a state in which one feels ever youthful, ever buoyant, and ever happy. Such a state is not only desirable but quite possible. And it is not only quite possible, it is easy to attain. This book will show you how you can attain perfect health and remain feeling ever youthful.

2

Ill Health

ANY DISCUSSION OF PERFECT HEALTH must include a few words about its very opposite, ill health. Below is a list of some of the most common problems encountered in everyday clinical practice. In the next few chapters I will talk about these specific problems of ill health. I will tell you how the medical community generally deals with them — this is the conventional approach, with which I sometimes agree — and I will tell you about my approach, which is unconventional at times and, I believe, sometimes more effective.

After dealing with these common problems, I devote the rest of the book to perfecting health and maintaining youthfulness. Then at the end of the book I build a case for the practice of a mental technique that makes all this possible. It is up to you the reader to decide for yourself whether the technique works or not, but you cannot decide this without trying it. If you are one of those people who is merely going to read this book without experiencing what it offers, then you are wasting your time. On the other hand, if you at least intend to try the suggestions, then read on — you have

perfect health and a feeling of everlasting youth to look forward
to.

But first let us turn to the problems of ill health and what the
conventional and unconventional thinking about them is. Here
are the sorts of patients I see in my medical practice every day:

1. People with hypertension, cardiovascular disease, and cere-
   brovascular disease, that is, high blood pressure, heart attack,
   and stroke
2. People with cancer
3. People with muscle aches and pains, arthritis, backache, and
   other musculoskeletal disorders
4. People with anxiety and depression, sleep disorders (primarily
   insomnia), and various psychological disorders
5. People suffering the effects of alcohol consumption, cigarette
   smoking, and drug abuse
6. People with weight problems, either too much or too little —
   usually too much; they complain, "I don't eat a thing, but I
   can't lose any weight."
7. People with fatigue for which no medical cause can be determined; they complain, "Why am I so tired all the time?"
8. People with various sexual problems
9. People suffering from stress and the "burned-out syndrome"
10. People with glandular problems, the most common being dia-
    betes
11. People with gastrointestinal problems, such as diarrhea,
    ulcers, and various complaints related to poor digestion
12. People suffering from various infections
13. People injured in household, automobile, or work-related ac-
    cidents

Now let us discuss these problems in detail, devoting more attention to the ones that are the most common causes of worry in
our society.

3

High Blood Pressure, Heart Attack, and Stroke

HYPERTENSION, or high blood pressure, is a very common disorder and affects a large proportion of the population. If you are thirty or over, you have at least a one in five chance of being hypertensive. What exactly is high blood pressure? Blood pressure is simply the pressure applied by the blood to the blood vessels as it passes through them. It is usually recorded in millimeters of mercury using an instrument called a sphygmomanometer, the familiar blood pressure cuff that inflates around the upper arm. The pressure recorded when the heart is contracting is called the systolic pressure — it should normally be less than 140 millimeters of mercury. The pressure recorded when the heart is relaxing is called the diastolic pressure — it should normally be less than 90 millimeters of mercury. In other words, normal blood pressure is said to be less than 140/90 (or "140 over 90"). Whenever blood pressure increases to more than 140/90, we call the condition hypertension, taking into account that blood pressure normally increases with age.

Hypertension is harmful and must be treated because it causes damage to vital organs, including the heart, kidneys, and brain.

Untreated, it leads to heart failure, stroke, and kidney failure, and consequently to a reduced life span. What is the cause of high blood pressure? In the vast majority of cases, medical researchers have been unable to find an exact cause for high blood pressure. Thus in more than 90 percent of the people with hypertension, no clear cause for the elevated blood pressure can be given.

A number of interesting observations have been made, however. First, there is evidence that abnormal psychological stimuli may play a role in the genesis of hypertension. Animals exposed experimentally to chronic stress can become hypertensive, and psychological stress is frequently seen in patients with hypertension. Moreover, sedatives and tranquilizers have been used successfully in the treatment of some kinds of hypertension. Most physicians therefore associate stress, and particularly psychological stress — even though it is to them a sort of "intangible tangible" — with hypertension. We will talk later about some of the personality factors most frequently seen in stressed people.

Another factor long implicated in the causation of high blood pressure is the intake of salt. People, as well as animals, can be made hypertensive by including a high intake of salt in their diet. (I devote all of chapter 6 to discussing the role of food in the cause and prevention of ill health since it is such a vital subject.)

Recently a great deal of interest has developed in the roles of hormones in hypertension. Hormones are chemicals produced by glandular structures in various parts of the body which have an effect on other parts of the body distant from the site where the hormones are produced. In other words, hormones are chemical messengers. Hormones that may be altered in cases of hypertension include cortisol, adrenaline, aldosterone, and renin. It is not really important for you to know these names or what these hormones do. The important fact is that the concentration of certain chemicals in the blood is altered in the person with hypertension. Hypertension caused by stress is actually thought to be mediated via these hormones — they are the tangible substances through which the intangible of "stress" affects the body. Doctors believe that such emotions as anxiety, fear, and anger cause an alteration

in certain chemicals in the brain. These chemicals, or neuro-
transmitters, as they are called, in turn can influence the secretion
of hormones such as ACTH from the pituitary, a gland located in
the head. These in their turn stimulate the adrenal glands located
over the kidneys, which then release hormones, such as cortisol
and adrenaline, into the blood, causing a rise in blood pressure.
This is only one example of a phenomenon that is being increasingly recognized as a key mechanism in the genesis of disease
processes. The phenomenon is the translation of an emotion or
thought into a chemical message, which in turn stimulates a distant organ. It is the first appearance of what I call the psychophysiological connection.

Since the consciousness of scientists and physicians is so di-
sease-oriented, most of the research so far has been conducted to
gain more understanding of disease-producing mechanisms. It
seems just as logical, however, for us to turn our attention in the
other direction and to say that positive emotions should have a
healthy, life-supporting influence on the body. In the foreseeable
future, biologists will be studying the alteration in neuro-transmitters that occurs when such positive thoughts as love, compassion, peace, courage, faith, and hope are introduced. What we
need to know more about is the exact pathway that a thought follows on its way to becoming a molecule in the body. A very important recent observation has been made showing that hormones
formerly thought to be present *only* in the blood stream have also
been discovered in significant concentrations in the brain tissue
itself. For example, renin, a hormone secreted by the kidneys and
implicated in organ damage that occurs in hypertension, is also
found in brain tissue. There it is associated with other hormones
and with the brain's own neuro-transmitters, the common ones
being dopamine, serotonin, epinephrine, and norepinephrine.
Leaving the names aside, these brain substances are just chemicals, ones that are closely associated with thoughts.

It is only a matter of time, then, before biologists will be able to
identify and demonstrate that changes in a person's thought patterns — perhaps a sudden upwelling of affection or the memory of

a loved family member — lead directly to changes in the levels of hormones and other chemicals in the brain and the cells of the body. In chapter 35 I will explore the simple and elegant technologies that already exist in this fascinating area of coordinating mind and body. We can actually use them to alter our thought patterns and emotions in a favorable direction and in that way directly affect the body in a favorable direction too.

Current Approaches to the Treatment of Hypertension — and Their Limitations

Drug Therapy

Most physicians use various kinds of drugs to treat hypertension. The reason for this is twofold. First, drugs are the quickest and easiest solution, both for the physician and for the patient. In an economy that is geared to productivity and at a time when the aim of physicians and people in general is to accomplish as much as possible with as little effort as possible, it is much easier for a physician to write a prescription than to sit down with a patient and go into all the reasons why he may be hypertensive and the changes in lifestyle that may be necessary to bring the blood pressure down. Moreover, in the majority of cases patients are not willing to change their lifestyles or their dietary habits. It is so much easier to swallow a pill, or a couple of pills, or, as we will see later, a lot of pills, and go about one's business.

The second reason why drugs are the most popular method of therapy for the treatment of hypertension is that they are effective, and some of them are very effective. We live in a society that demands instant solutions to all problems, no matter what the expense. The pharmaceutical industry, backed by the scientific community at large, has spent years and years of research and billions of dollars to develop some of their most effective pharmaceutical agents to apply to the treatment of hypertension. If pills are so effective and so easy to take, then what is the problem?

Drug therapy has its problems and limitations:

1. Drugs are expensive. The cost of research into finding better products is of course passed on to the consumer. Some antihypertensive agents these days cost up to a dollar a pill, and a pill may have to be taken several times a day, sometimes for life.

2. All drugs, without exception, have side effects. There is no such thing as a perfect pill. Some of the common side effects associated with antihypertensive agents make quite a list, including fatigue, dryness of the mouth, blurred vision, disturbance of taste, sexual dysfunction (often in the form of impotence in men), dizziness, lack of concentration and memory, damage to the liver, kidneys, or bone marrow, and a range of emotional disturbances from irritability to severe depression. The list becomes longer still when you consider less common but still observed side effects. Many patients learn to live with some of the less serious, or relatively "minor" side effects, such as a little fatigue (all the time) and dryness of the mouth. A number of people, however, refuse to take a medicine because they cannot tolerate its side effects, even though they realize that their hypertension may be life threatening and will almost surely shorten their life span. In medical parlance such refusal on the part of patients is called noncompliance, and although it is often considered out of the physician's hands, in fact noncompliance is one of the major problems in the treatment of hypertension.

3. Drugs have to be taken for a lifetime since they are not really a cure, and people hate the idea of being dependent on something for the rest of their lives. (One finds this a major problem in treating every disease, such as diabetes or glaucoma, when patients are instructed to take their medication every day for life.)

4. Drug tolerance, or tachyphylaxis, becomes a problem over time. It is a frequently observed phenomenon in biology and is said to occur when continued use of a drug ceases to be effective or when larger doses are required to produce the same effect. Frequently in the treatment of hypertension a drug will no longer be effective after continued use, and producing the desired biological

result calls for larger dosages, with the likelihood of course that side effects will also increase.

So we see that there are several disadvantages to the treatment of high blood pressure with drugs. What are some of the non-pharmacological approaches to the treatment of hypertension?

Hypertension Diets

The connection between high blood pressure and too much salt in the diet, which I have already mentioned, has been well documented. Lowering salt intake in the diet, frequently to the point of adding no salt at all to one's food, proves an effective means of lowering blood pressure, particularly if the blood pressure is only moderately elevated. Most physicians caution their patients against excessive salt intake, but since dietary habits are ingrained over a lifetime, many patients find it very difficult to follow even this proven recommendation.

Other parts of our ordinary diet have also been implicated as possible causes of high blood pressure. Among the most suspect are: (1) the large amount of saturated fat found in any diet containing butter, cream, and large quantities of meat; (2) the addition of the hormone estrogen and related chemicals, which has become standard practice in the cattle feed industry; and (3) the lack of dietary fiber in any diet that depends upon processed food rather than whole grains, fruits, and vegetables. For patients willing to change their habits, numerous dietary approaches to hypertension now exist. The proponents of the Pritikin diet and macrobiotics are particularly visible, but in a less publicized way many forward-looking physicians and medical institutions have adopted similar dietary treatments. The basic tactic in all these diets is to decrease salt, animal fats, whole milk, and refined starches and sugar in favor of poultry and fish, skim milk, whole grains, and fiber-rich fruits and vegetables. Since our bad dietary habits have been linked to almost every one of the so-called life-style diseases that plague affluent societies around the world, such diets can naturally be effective, particularly in mild to moderate cases of hypertension.

All special diets, however, have the same drawback — patients find it very difficult to stay on such diets, even when they realize that it is medically imperative for them to do so. Eating, which should be pleasurable and natural, falls into the category of "doctor's orders," and over each meal hangs the threat of damaging one's health if some dish is too good to resist. Patients are not simply being foolish here, because in a deeper sense it is not healthy at all to approach eating in a mood of tension, strain, and self-consciousness. Although cases of existing hypertension certainly call for a sensible, controlled therapeutic diet, what is needed even more is a return to the state in which the body can be trusted to eat the right food in the first place. The basic premise we want to live by is that our bodies know what is good for them. In order to live that way, we need a technique that will cultivate right habits and eliminate wrong ones spontaneously. The patient needs to change without being aware of change, and that means that the approach must be at a level deeper than that of good intentions.

Mental Techniques

Are mental techniques the answer, then? Several approaches have in recent years been popularized in the treatment of hypertension. Among the most notable ones are biofeedback, various kinds of relaxation, visualization techniques, and meditation.

Biofeedback: In this technique the patient is outfitted with a device on the arm that monitors his blood pressure. On an instrument panel he can view the fluctuations in blood pressure as they occur spontaneously. He can then teach himself either to raise or lower his blood pressure by simply willing or desiring it to fluctuate in either direction. From the continuous feedback he obtains from the instrument panel, the patient is learning to affect a bodily function that is normally autonomic, that is, spontaneously self-regulated without the need of our attention. This is a clear example of how medicine is making use of the psychophysiological connection — a desire is being channeled into a physiological response.

In practice, however, biofeedback as it is currently available is not a very effective means of controlling moderately severe hypertension. Yet the simple, demonstrated fact that a person can change his blood pressure simply by desiring to do so is in itself a fascinating and extremely important observation. It establishes yet another example of how thoughts translate themselves into physiological effects. Everyone is familiar with the way that erotic feelings or fearful thoughts or excited emotions immediately arouse the body, and at times with uncanny speed and power; therefore, it should be no surprise that a much greater range of thoughts and emotions can provoke other physiological responses, even at the body's subtlest levels. It may be that biofeedback has been disappointing because the patient is too dependent upon the machine — he is trying to induce by artificial means what he could learn to do better by contacting a deeper source within himself. The key thing to learn from the studies on biofeedback is that we can change our blood pressure, or any autonomic function, by changing our thought patterns.

Relaxation: Because of interest in stress management, a large market exists for relaxation techniques. Some of these techniques work on the gross level by manipulating the body directly, others employ a sequence of relaxing exercises combined with calming thoughts or suggestions, while still others rely on the body's innate ability to relax when put into a suitable frame of mind (popularized as the "relaxation response"). Some of these have proved effective in the treatment of high blood pressure, but their usefulness is limited at the moment to treating mild hypertension. Often this approach has the same drawback as biofeedback: the technique lowers blood pressure while it is being practiced, but the beneficial effects do not linger afterward or they fail to offset the results of tense situations that cause blood pressure to elevate suddenly and, for some people, to remain elevated. Also, since any relaxation technique must be followed faithfully and be practiced every day, sometimes several times a day, many people find that sheer boredom prevents them from carrying out the program.

Visualization: This is a variation on the relaxation techniques that works directly through the mind. The subject is asked to visualize, with his eyes closed, a calm and serene picture. Visualization has the advantage of being usable at any time and in any place. As a technique it has been shown useful in cases of mild hypertension.

Meditation: Long-term studies have proved that meditation, if regularly kept up, effectively reduces high blood pressure. The variable results found in some studies may stem from the notion, common in medical circles, that all forms of meditation are alike. In my experience, by far the most promising meditation technique is Transcendental Meditation, or TM. It also happens to be the easiest and most widely practiced meditation technique in the country. People who practice the TM technique on a regular basis do not develop hypertension. Compared with relaxation techniques, Transcendental Meditation shows more cumulative and lasting results — lowered blood pressure continues outside the actual time of meditation — and people are happy to stay with it for years on end. Clearly, correct meditation acts from a very deep level within ourselves, so I will return to the subject for longer discussion after developing the whole theme of the psychophysiological connection.

General Prevention

Since the cause of hypertension is not known in most cases, no exact method of prevention has been determined. However, it is well known that certain risk factors lead to a higher chance of developing high blood pressure. If you are more than a few pounds overweight, if you smoke, if you take no regular exercise, or if there is a history of hypertension in your family, then you are considered to be at a higher risk for developing high blood pressure. Treatment regimens that have patients lose weight, stop smoking, and perform aerobic exercise on a regular basis have proved quite effective in reducing hypertension. Once again, however, it becomes a matter of what lifestyle changes a person is willing to make and can keep up for the rest of his life.

In this section I have sketched the current views on the causes, consequences, and treatment for hypertension. Clearly, most of the approaches are not ideal. As part of any attempt to lead a normal, spontaneous life, some are very far from ideal. What is the answer? Is there some means by which we can prevent hypertension from occurring and cure it once it has occurred? I believe that the key lies in a better understanding of ourselves. For that, we will first have to understand what we mean by "ourselves." Who or what is the "self"? A clearer answer will begin to appear as we continue to describe the state of health at its deepest level.

Heart Disease and Heart Attacks

Coronary artery disease is the number one killer in the United States and in the rest of the Western world. The disease involves hardening of the coronary arteries, the blood vessels that carry oxygen to the heart. When they become blocked by hardened deposits of plaque, the heart muscle is deprived of oxygen, and this results in the death of heart muscle, or myocardial infarction (the common medical term for heart attack). A severe heart attack of course results in death, usually within a few hours of onset. What are the most common risk factors associated with heart attack?

1. Obesity: fat people are more likely to suffer a heart attack than thin people.

2. High blood pressure: I have discussed this serious risk factor at some length in the preceding section.

3. Stress: psychological stress is considered a significant risk factor in heart disease. Some authorities even profile a particular type of personality, called a Type A, that is more prone than normal to coronary artery disease. Type A people (usually men) are aggressive, impatient, tense, and hard driving. Forever trying to beat a deadline and unable to allow themselves to relax, their primary sickness is that of being always in a hurry. Medical re-

searchers have questioned whether there actually exists a clear-cut Type A personality, but there is no doubt that hostility or fear or any powerful enough psychological stress can contribute to heart disease. (For a dramatic case in which such emotions led directly to a heart attack, see chapter 13.)

4. Increased cholesterol: high levels of cholesterol in the blood, or hypercholesterolemia, is found more frequently than normal in people with coronary artery disease. Cholesterol is a fatty chemical, or lipid, that is found in certain foods as well as in our blood. People who eat a lot of cholesterol-rich food, such as eggs and red meat, tend to develop increased cholesterol in their blood, so evidently this risk is directly related to diet. Research has proved that eating a great deal of rich food in general increases the risk of hardening of the blood vessels.

5. Smoking: smokers are much more likely to suffer from heart attacks (and cancer) than nonsmokers. Take just three risk factors — high blood pressure, high blood cholesterol, and smoking; the chances of a heart attack are nearly doubled if any one of them is present in a person's medical profile, quadrupled if two are present, and multiplied eightfold if all three are found.

6. Lack of physical exercise: heart attacks occur more frequently among inactive people and among those who lead mostly sedentary lives.

7. Other more specific risk factors include genetics — your risk is higher if there is already a family history of heart attacks — uncontrolled diabetes, and old age. Being born a male has always been a classic risk factor too, but this is slowly changing as women expose themselves to the privileges of a man's world, such as smoking, obesity, inactivity, and Type A tensions.

It is obvious from this list that most of these risk factors are under our control. We can control obesity, smoking, lack of exercise, stress, and to a great extent high blood pressure. Coronary artery disease therefore seems preventable. Yet its levels are only slowly declining in our society. Why is it that some of us are successful at controlling risk factors and some are not so successful? Again, I think the answer will emerge only through a better understanding of ourselves, in discovering exactly what this "self" is that holds the key to self-control — not the superficial, damaging self-control of a Type A, but the assured, spontaneous, relaxed self-control that is part of perfect health.

Stroke

The same hardening and deterioration of blood vessels that causes heart attacks also causes strokes, but in this case the affected area is the brain. Stroke occurs when one of the blood vessels leading to the brain is blocked or ruptured. The severity of the resulting damage to the brain depends upon how serious the blockage or bleeding has been. Mild strokes may result in muscle weakness, blurred vision, unclear speech, and other defects in the senses. Severe strokes lead to paralysis or death.

Once a person has suffered a stroke, the only possible treatment is physical therapy to restore the impaired or lost functions. Despite great progress in this kind of treatment, full recovery from a serious stroke is rare. The only sensible approach is prevention.

The causes of stroke are tied to illness of the cardiovascular system in general, so the earlier section on heart disease applies to stroke as well. Once again, smoking, hypertension, old age, and a family history of strokes create particularly high risks, but any factor that contributes to atherosclerosis, or blockage of the arteries by fat deposits, also poses the danger of stroke.

4

Cancer

CANCER IS THE TERM used to define an abnormal growth of cells in the body. The abnormal cells invade normal tissue and spread to other organs, causing improper functioning and finally death to those organs. It is estimated that one out of four Americans will develop some sort of cancer during his lifetime. Although the exact cause of cancer at the molecular level has not yet been defined, it is generally agreed that there are many different kinds of cancer and that certain outside agents are identifiable as causes of specific cancers.

Causes of Cancer

Viruses: It is now fairly well established that certain viruses can cause cancer. For example, EB virus, which is usually the infectious agent in the common disease infectious mononucleosis (popularly called "mono"), has been shown to cause Burkitt's lymphoma, a specific cancer of the lymph glands. It is also a cause of nasopharyngeal cancer, which affects the nose and the cavity between the mouth and esophagus. Obviously, all people who get mononucleosis do not develop cancer. In fact, only a small or even a minute proportion of the people who are exposed to this virus will develop cancer. Why is it that a virus will cause cancer in some people and not in others? The exact reason is not known. However, it seems that some people are more prone to contracting a disease of any kind, including cancer.

A number of host factors are involved in this, including a condition called immunosuppression. This term denotes decreased immunity, or a loss in the body's ability to fight a disease, usually an infection or cancer. What can bring about immunosuppression? Several factors are implicated, including viruses, drug use, and poor nutrition. In some cases, immunosuppression occurs because the body produces the wrong kinds of antibodies, which fail to distinguish between harmful outside agents and the body's own cells. When this happens and the body's defense mechanisms cannot tell what is "self" and what is "nonself," then resistance to invading organisms decreases, and infection or cancer may then result. Whatever the causes for this at the cellular or chemical level, we are seeing once again that our understanding of the "self" is vitally important.

Carcinogens: A number of cancer-causing agents, or carcinogens, have been isolated in certain foods, in the work environment of certain occupations, and in specific chemicals. A list of the best-proved ones includes:

1. Tobacco smoke, which is linked to lung cancer, mouth cancer, bronchial cancer, and associated with bladder cancer
2. Asbestos, which is known to cause lung cancer
3. Vinyl chloride, a cause of liver cancer
4. Uranium, which is linked to lung cancer
5. Naphthalene dyes, known to cause bladder cancer
6. Nitrates and nitrites of the kind used routinely to preserve meats, which are strongly implicated in stomach and intestinal cancer

Certain hormones and drugs, including some used to treat cancer, can also cause cancer. Exposure to nuclear radiation, to too much sunlight, or to excessive x-rays are known causes of cancer, as are a host of industrial agents from common chimney soot to arsenic, coal tars, and dry-cleaning fluid. Carcinogens in combination make the risk of cancer even higher; in particular, tobacco smoke and asbestos greatly increase the danger from other carcinogens and from each other.

In addition to these proven carcinogens, quite a few foods are linked to cancer strongly enough to make them very suspect. In fact, cancer is coming to be seen more and more as a lifestyle disease that can be prevented by changing our habits, and so increased attention is being paid to the kind of diet that might reduce the risk of developing cancer. See the later section in this chapter where I discuss this important approach in some detail.

Other possible causes: People likely to develop cancer may have inherited that tendency, though the exact mechanism is not yet known. Through their DNA, all cells inherit their ability to reproduce normally. When this self-regulated ability is lost and a cell begins to multiply itself out of control, it is in effect fathering its own line of "immortal" cells. At the heart of the cell some bit of the genetic code has developed into an oncogene, or cancer gene. Such a cell wildly and uselessly reproduces itself, destroying other cells that are useful. In general, this mechanism is now well understood. The problem is how to connect a process at the level of the genes with the larger environment of air, water, food, and inherited qualities.

Stress is of great interest for the role it may play in the development of cancer. In some quite powerful, direct way our cells are able to react to stress. Stress is internal, not external, as people commonly think. A perception of an outside demand by the brain or any particular part of the body is the actual stress — it is a response of some kind. As the result of a stress response, changes occur in the musculoskeletal system, the nervous system, the endocrine system (responsible for important hormones), and the immune system. How stress is related to cancer is not exactly known. Current theories hold that stress triggers the release of hormones from the pituitary, such as ACTH, which then cause the release of another hormone, cortisol, from the adrenal glands. Cortisol is known to decrease the body's immunity to disease because it inhibits the production of antibodies and "killer" T-cells, cells produced by the thymus gland that are responsible for disease surveillance in the immune system. The overall result when we follow this chain of events from a stress to a decrease in immune response is that the body becomes more susceptible, so researchers suspect, to viruses and carcinogens.

At a more general level, from simply observing their patients, some doctors believe that there is a definite link between psychological stress and developing cancer. Whether or not cancer is caused by the presence of "stress hormones" in the blood, it seems significant that the disease strikes single, widowed, and divorced people more often than those who are married, and stress is known to be higher in single people. The personality profiles of cancer patients may also show that these people have a tendency to bottle up strong emotions and to take a habitual stance of not allowing themselves free expression in life. Somehow an inner environment that is keyed up by stress and has no viable outlet tends a person toward cancer. I find this very important when thinking about a strategy for preventing cancer.

Current Approaches to the Treatment of Cancer

No completely satisfactory treatment exists. The current options are:

Surgery: If the cancerous tumor is restricted to one organ or to only a portion of it, then sometimes a cure can be effected by removing the organ or the diseased portion of it. This happens only rarely. The surgical procedure is often mutilating, a great source of distress to patients, and can result in severe disabilities because a functioning organ has been taken from the body.

Radiation: Some cancer cells will die when exposed to radiation or x-rays in high doses. The problem of course is that radiation will also damage normal, healthy cells at the same time. The treatment can cause devastating side effects and debility in the patient, who will feel very weak and sick. In general, radiation will not actually cure cancer.

Chemotherapy: Treatment with drugs, or chemotherapy, is effective in a number of cancers. The medications are often associated, however, with very debilitating and devastating side effects, among them hair loss, impotence, sterility, nausea, and vomiting. By causing immunosuppression, which we have already discussed, chemotherapy can also make the patient more susceptible to other types of cancer.

Mental Techniques and Spontaneous Remission of Cancer

Medical research is learning more and more about the mind-body connection in various diseases, and cancer is no exception. A rare but well-known phenomenon among cancer patients is "spontaneous remission," that is, complete recovery from cancer for no known reason. Physicians who regularly treat cancer patients know very well that the ones who have a strong, positive attitude do much better than those with a negative attitude, who face their cancer feeling only helplessness and despair.

In a study reported by cancer specialist Dr. Carl Simonton in 1975, the attitudes and course of treatment for 152 cancer patients were examined together. The response to treatment was ranked from excellent to poor for each patient. Twenty patients showed excellent response to their treatments. All twenty of these patients also displayed what was described as a positive attitude. Fourteen of them were in very poor condition at the outset and would have had less than a 50 percent chance of surviving five years, according to all available statistics.

Twenty-two patients did extremely poorly in the course of treatment. All of them, moreover, showed negative attitudes about their situation. These positive or negative attitudes are basically extensions of positive or negative thought processes. Positive attitudes generate the powerful emotions of faith, hope, courage, happiness, and belief. At the other extreme, negative attitudes generate feelings of fear, hostility, helplessness, and despair, which are equally powerful. So attitude is not something to consider superficially; the difference between positive and negative attitudes, so far as they affect the body's ability to survive a crisis, is like having two different diseases. One we pronounce curable, the other incurable.

Can positive attitudes be created, or do they already have to exist by nature? Various mental techniques, including visualization therapies, are showing promise as useful additions to the treatment of cancer. In one approach, patients are asked to visualize their disease, their treatment, and the body's defenses by forming concrete images of their own. Some see battles in space, others picture flowing masses of light and dark. I had a fascinating encounter with such a technique. I saw a patient who had come to my office for a physical exam. She was a vigorous-looking young woman, extremely bright and appealing, who needed the physical as part of a job application.

While working up her medical history, I discovered that this patient had once been diagnosed as having non–Hodgkin's lymphoma, a cancer of the lymph glands. She had been advised to seek treatment at one of the prominent teaching hospitals associated with a famous medical school in the Boston area. There she received the initial course of chemotherapy. Her cancer was extremely far advanced, being described as a Stage IV B, which meant that it included invasion of the bone marrow. The patient suffered extremely debilitating side effects from the chemotherapy and decided not to finish the full course of her treatment. Both her father and mother were physicians, and she was under intense pressure from her whole family to continue with this treatment.

Rather than endure the pressure, she left the country to live in a small European town for a year. There she practiced on her own, after reading a great deal about them, the simple visualization techniques proposed by Dr. Simonton. A year later she returned to Boston. She had noticed that her swollen lymph nodes and the abnormal masses in various parts of her body had spontaneously diminished in size. When she was seen again at the cancer clinic of the same hospital where she had previously been examined, all the physicians were extremely puzzled at the complete absence of any evidence that this patient had cancer.

They asked her what kind of chemotherapy she had been receiving and where she had received it. When she told them that she had not undergone any additional standard medical treatment but had been practicing the Simonton technique entirely on her own, the doctors' reaction was typical of the medical establishment in general. They told her that her recovery was known as a spontaneous remission, but they did not discuss it further, explore it with her, or even inform her what a spontaneous remission was. In their minds the term itself, spontaneous remission, allowed them to dismiss the phenomenon. Like many scientists and physicians, they had closed minds. In actual fact, this patient had been practicing a definite technique, and in her mind at least, there was a cause-and-effect relationship between the technique and the clinical results that ensued.

In another, recent instance I had a patient with lung cancer who showed an unusually good response to radiation and chemotherapy. She confided to me two years after she was cured that every morning she would sit down with her eyes closed and repeat to herself for about ten minutes, "I am going to get better, I am going to recover completely." She said that she sincerely believed that this would happen and had absolute faith in her affirmations. She repeated this procedure four or five times a day but did not reveal what she was doing to anyone at the time, including me. Only several years afterward did she let out her secret. Now, three years after her initial treatment, she shows no clinical evidence of the lung cancer.

Since then, I have mentioned these examples to several of my patients, counseling them to keep the fact that they are practicing such techniques in strict secrecy and not to speak of it to anyone. This is because I feared that negative comments from friends and family might diminish the effectiveness of the practice. I am convinced from my observation of these patients so far that they are doing much better than they would have otherwise. I also strongly recommend that they pursue radiation therapy, chemotherapy, or surgery if it is considered necessary by an oncologist, a cancer specialist, but I believe that mental techniques play an important supporting role in their treatment, at the very least.

I am strongly convinced that one can isolate a typical kind of person who gets cancer, but at the same time I believe that cancer can be overcome, that it can be prevented as well as cured by establishing the right mental attitude. We have already seen that cancer cells, in their mindless, useless multiplication, have lost touch with their basic intelligence, the know-how at the genetic level that should regulate proper cell division. Somehow these mental techniques restore intelligence by operating from the mind's awareness. It is one intelligence in our bodies speaking to another and bringing it back to normal. What seems so promising is that the cure grows from within the patient, taking advantage of the mind-body connection.

The Role of Diet in Cancer, or the Diet-Cancer Connection

Although outspoken members of the lay public have often declared that there is a connection between cancer and the food we eat, the medical establishment, in fact the scientific community at large, was once very slow to study and establish the diet-cancer connection. Recently, however, a great many scientists have come to believe that the connection exists. The National Research Council has now issued a report entitled *Diet, Nutrition, and Cancer* (1983). It represents the most comprehensive review yet of the worldwide research on diet and cancer, but with the customary caution that the evidence for the link between them is still incomplete. Nevertheless, the council has issued the following dietary guidelines as a means of helping to prevent cancer:

1. Fats should be considerably reduced in the daily diet. For a typical American, fat consumption amounts to roughly 40–45 percent of the calories in a day's food intake. The report recommends reducing this to 30 percent, which for many people means cutting the amount of fatty foods by half. The council observes

that the association of fat intake with certain types of cancer, particularly of the breast, colon, and prostate, represents the strongest cause-and-effect relationship in the entire field of diet and cancer. These types of cancer are major killers in our society.

2. More whole-grain cereals, fresh fruit, and vegetables should be eaten, particularly those high in vitamin C. The council also recommends concentrating on fruits and vegetables that are high in beta-carotene (an organic chemical the body converts to vitamin A). These include dark green leafy vegetables, carrots, squash, and all relatives of cabbage, such as broccoli, brussels sprouts, and cauliflower.

3. Very little of salt-cured, pickled, or smoked foods should be consumed. These include sausage, bacon, hot dogs, smoked fish, and ham. The council has not yet recommended an entirely meatless diet, but I will present the arguments for that later on.

4. Alcohol should be consumed only in moderation. In making this recommendation the council points to the strong association between alcohol and cancers of the mouth, esophagus, and stomach. The council is being very cautious here in still allowing any alcohol at all. I believe that alcohol in any amount predisposes the drinker to a higher risk of cancer.

5. High-dose vitamin supplements, well over the government's recommended daily allowance (RDA), should be avoided. The rationale here is that toxicity can result from large doses of certain vitamins, particularly vitamins A and E. However, doctors rarely see such toxicity among their patients, and in my view supplemental vitamins have a beneficial effect. For instance, vitamins A, C, and E probably play a role in preventing cancer, although the optimal doses for this purpose have not been determined. Vitamins C and E act as antioxidants, which detoxify certain carcinogens. Vitamin A helps in inhibiting certain precancerous changes in cell membranes.

I routinely make the following additional recommendations to my patients regarding diet, daily habits, and cancer:

1. Don't smoke. In addition to directly causing lung cancer, to-

bacco smoke increases the likelihood that other carcinogens in the air will cause this disease, including substances that on their own would not be cancer producing.

2. Don't overeat. Obesity is linked to a high incidence of certain cancers, particularly of the uterus and kidneys.

3. Don't drink alcohol, even in moderation.

4. Avoid excesses of hot coffee, tea, and cola drinks. Excessive drinking of hot tea has been linked to stomach cancer in Japan. There appears to be a higher incidence of cancer of the pancreas among heavy coffee drinkers — this means more than three cups per day. Tea, coffee, chocolate, and cola drinks are heavy in substances called methylxanthines. These may be suspect because they stimulate certain cell reactions that make the cells sensitive to particular hormones, although the implications are not fully understood. I advise caution nonetheless.

5. Include generous amounts of roughage and fibrous foods in the diet. There is a correlation between colon cancer and low fiber in the Western diet. Adding fiber from whole grains, fruits, and vegetables perhaps serves to buffer potential carcinogens when they are passing through the intestines during digestion; in any case, people who eat a high-fiber diet have lower risk of developing colon cancer.

6. Avoid charcoal-grilled meat and fish, or any burned food. It has been quite conclusively demonstrated that charcoal grilling produces carcinogens from charred fats.

7. Take supplemental vitamins if the diet is poor in vitamins A, C, and E.

8. Avoid all moldy or stale foods. Molds are known to produce carcinogens.

9. Don't limit your diet to the same few foods repeated over and over. Variety in diet is likely to prevent the intake of too much of any single carcinogen, including the natural carcinogens that various vegetables appear to produce to ward off insects and fungus, although this area is still quite obscure to researchers.

10. Eat a generally well-balanced diet, taking all foods in mod-

eration and as much as possible drinking pure water — the problem of industrial toxins appearing in our drinking water has become a serious concern in many parts of the country.

Additional recommendations will be found in chapter 26, "Diet and Destiny," but we can already see that if cancer is to be prevented, the dietary approach is much the same, so far as the general points go, as for the other lifestyle diseases. Moreover, we can see that the huge number of isolated factors that contribute to cancer can be divided into two broad categories:

1. Outside agents, including viruses, carcinogens, and suspect influences from the environment, and

2. Intrinsic problems with the host, that is, the person who develops cancer. It is these that give rise to a susceptibility to cancer in the body itself. By and large almost all cancers should theoretically be preventable if we avoid exposing ourselves to the causative agents (although excluding all of them is clearly out of our control) and if we decrease our susceptibility in the first place. This means finding a means, if there is one, of promoting the body's own inner resistance to cancer-causing agents. Ultimately, what we already know about cancer is leading us deeper in our search for the psychophysiological connection.

5

Cigarette Smoking,
Alcohol, and Drug Abuse

IF CIGARETTES, alcohol, and "recreational" drugs were eliminated from society, we would have nearly empty hospitals. A large percentage of patients admitted to a hospital for illness can trace the origins of their disease, or the conditions that aggravate it, back to smoking, drinking, indulging in recreational marijuana or stronger drugs, and sometimes to a combination of all three. I will talk briefly about the danger to health that they represent, but we are all aware that smoking, drinking, and drug abuse receive very little support in our society. Warnings, good intentions, and even public awareness campaigns do not do much good here. The important question, then, is what it really takes to stop these obviously threatening abuses.

Cigarette Smoking

More than seventy million Americans smoke, and the reason they do is that they are habituated — many physicians would say addicted — to nicotine. Nicotine is a poison that the body can get used to, as it gets used to alcohol. Once the body gets over its initial dislike of nicotine, then the "pleasurable" effects of smoking support the habit. These pleasures are largely in the mind — the smoker looks on cigarettes as either a stimulant or a relaxant, depending on what he mentally needs.

Smoking is undoubtedly a significant contributor to our two major killers, heart disease and cancer. Coronary artery disease is fifty times more common in smokers than in nonsmokers. Compared with nonsmokers, people who smoke one pack of cigarettes a day are eight times more likely to contract lung cancer. This likelihood increases to eighteen times if between one and two packs a day are smoked, and to twenty-one times if a person smokes more than two packs a day. The actual death rate for smokers is 70 percent higher from coronary artery disease, 500 percent higher from bronchitis and cancer, and 1,000 percent higher from lung cancer than it is for nonsmokers. Smokers are far more likely to develop other diseases of all kinds, among them emphysema, ulcers, and cancers of the mouth, esophagus, stomach, and bladder. So-called low-tar cigarettes often contain higher quantities of other toxins, and low-nicotine cigarettes in general usually lead smokers merely to smoke more packs a day.

Without question, smoking is a disease and warrants immediate medical attention. All sorts of programs to help people to quit smoking have been put forward, and almost all can be effective. The group programs sponsored by the American Cancer Society and various hospitals have had notable success. These groups offer the sympathetic support of other smokers who are trying to quit, and this is a great help when anyone suffers the real and sometimes prolonged withdrawal symptoms of nicotine addiction. Studies have shown that no single method is the key. Those people who have stopped successfully usually try several times, using a variety of approaches, before they become entirely free of their habit.

I believe that smoking ends with a single "mutation" in the brain that offers the thought, "I have no desire for this anymore." With this insight comes the spontaneous realization that "I can quit, it is easy for me." In other words, it is not really the treatment that is working — rather, it is the newfound attitude that there is no problem in the first place. When this insight is allowed to enter the mind, then any treatment will work, including simply stopping.

By promoting the thought that smoking is difficult to stop and by backing this up with detailed descriptions of the physical addictiveness of nicotine, doctors in fact are making it difficult for people to quit. They are helping a wrong attitude, a wrong reality view, to sink its roots into the minds of their patients. This helps explain, I think, why people continue to harm themselves by smoking even though they are aware of the danger they face. The willingness to stop comes when the idea of danger is *not* present.

Alcohol

No one any longer argues with the fact that alcoholism is a disease. Alcoholics are subject to distinctly higher than average death rates (these rates increase even more if they are also smokers). People with a history of heavy drinking experience a death rate three times that of nondrinkers. Their deaths are commonly caused by diseases of the digestive system, suicide, automobile accidents, and malnutrition. Destruction of heart muscle, brain tissue, liver, pancreas, and stomach occurs frequently as well.

When it comes to occasional drinking of alcohol, however, society and the medical profession tend to display a different attitude. Some physicians have gone so far as to suggest that small amounts of alcohol may even have beneficial effects. By this they usually mean that one drink, say a glass of wine, temporarily lowers blood pressure and releases inhibitions and worries. It is interesting to note that in a survey in which people were asked, "What constitutes excessive alcohol consumption?" the definition of "excessive" was whatever exceeded the respondent's own intake.

I believe that alcohol is a toxin. It impairs clear perception and motor coordination. It has poisonous effects on the heart, liver, and brain that do not seem to be reversible. It contributes to senseless deaths from automobile accidents that number twenty-five thousand fatalities a year. Anything that harmful, even in small doses, is not a legitimate part of perfect health; therefore, I recommend complete abstinence from alcohol.

What causes alcohol addiction in the first place? Some people may be predisposed to alcoholism, either by heredity or by family upbringing. Identical twins who have been separated at infancy and raised apart have been shown to develop similar drinking habits after they grow up, and if one becomes an alcoholic, the other tends to at around the same time. Other people tend to drift slowly but steadily into alcoholism, starting with occasional drinking in adolescence. I think it is significant that both drinking and smoking begin in the teenage years for most people, at a time when the self is confused and unformed. This helps both habits to become ingrained at a deep level of the personality and makes it difficult for healthy adult thought patterns to displace the established mindset. As with smoking, the treatment for alcoholism requires a single, deep-seated change in attitude. Successful group programs like Alcoholics Anonymous offer support to make this inner change come about. Without it, no change is really possible.

Recreational Drugs

The term *recreational drugs* loosely includes all the various substances people take to enhance, distort, or otherwise affect perception. A person initially resorts to using such drugs because the experience with them is pleasurable. In our society the range of pleasures can be derived from many sources, mainly alcohol, opiates (morphine, codeine, heroin), marijuana, cocaine, and various hallucinogens like mescaline and LSD. But an enormous list could be gathered of substances that alter brain chemistry and therefore could be said to affect the mind. People opposed to the use of coffee, tea, and even sugar may with some reason label them drugs.

In the last decade, scientists were fascinated to discover that the human brain is capable of synthesizing chemicals very similar to opiates. They named these endorphins, from *end-,* which means from within the body, and *orphin,* which has the same root as morphine. These "endogenous opiates" are the body's own pain relievers and in fact prove to be much more powerful than pain-killers you can buy in a drugstore. Recent investigation has also shown that the brain possesses distinct receptor cells for receiving these endorphins. An opiate we might be given from outside (called an "exogenous opiate") exerts its painkilling effect on the brain by binding to these same receptors. That such receptors have evolved at all means that there must be some use for them; the inner and outer opiates seem to serve the same function just because they fit into the same receptors.

Yet the brain can also be affected by the entire list of drugs given at first, including very powerful, mind-altering hallucinogens. The implication is that receptors must exist in the brain for these too, or for their analogues (their chemical equivalents). In other words, we must be capable of synthesizing such drugs or their analogues inside ourselves, to an extent at least; otherwise, why would we have evolved the receptors to bind them? This conclusion offers a clue to the perplexing question of why people have sought and experimented with mind-altering drugs since time immemorial.

Perhaps the human organism is meant to experience a wider range of consciousness than we suppose. Mind-altering drugs apparently work at all because our internal system of receptors and analogues is already available. What is unclear now is exactly what natural, healthy condition of mind and body would induce altered states as a normal part of life. It may be that when our quota of these states is not ordinarily fulfilled, we tend to fill the gap with analogues from the outside.

However, the pharmacological analogues, not having been designed for us spontaneously by our body's innate wisdom, have their toxicity. The recent increased use of these drugs has brought to light the fact that toxicity accompanies almost every one of them. For example, marijuana was thought until recently to be relatively safe but now has been shown to affect unfavorably the immune system. The principal active ingredient in marijuana (THC) localizes in high concentration in the spleen, among other places. The spleen is an important site for the manufacture of T-lymphocytes, a specialized part of the immune system important in fighting off cancer as well as various infections. The T-lymphocytes in the bodies of regular marijuana smokers fight against disease less well than normally. Not only are fewer T-lymphocytes present, but they are also sluggish and slower to divide when faced with an enemy force, namely, potential infection.

Data on the impairment of the immune system from the habitual use of marijuana has not received the publicity it deserves. In a significant finding by one Columbia University study, the antibodies produced by marijuana smokers declined drastically during one month of heavy use. When smoking was totally discontinued, however, the antibodies only returned to normal levels very slowly, and even five weeks later there were signs of a decrease. Although this finding of immunotoxicity (damage to the immune system) is most striking in the case of marijuana, it is apparently induced by other drug addictions as well. Unless attitudes toward drug taking change significantly, we face the prospect of large numbers of people who use recreational drugs becoming highly susceptible to disease.

These drugs are also harmful just because they do alter the mind by directly acting on brain tissue. Simply from daily observation, one commonly sees that the euphoria induced by drugs in time changes to something quite different. Drug users of all types not only tend to addiction and require larger and larger doses to satisfy their urges, but the actual effect of the drug on the brain changes. Pleasant sensations give way to lethargy, withdrawal, depression, dullness, and other psychologically damaging states. Sometimes physicians refer to these as "underlying states of mind," but it is just as likely that continued use has in fact altered the structure of brain tissue. The brain centers responsible for emotions and biological rhythms are stimulated by many recreational drugs, and there is evidence that this artificial enhancement leads to some sort of overtaxing, or burnout, with the sad consequences we all observe in our society.

I don't need to belabor the point that drug taking does great harm to young people, making the difficult transition to adulthood even more difficult and almost wrenching. And drugs obviously contribute directly to crime, accidents, suicide, and murder. Achieving a natural, beneficial enhancement of consciousness can be a great stride forward in personal development, as we shall see. Drugs may imitate such a state for a little while, but in truth they are its enemies.

Smoking, drinking, and drug abuse exist because they satisfy a natural need that has become a craving. To solve the problems they create, we must look once again to the human mind. Why do some people crave mind-altering stimuli? Can we substitute other stimuli — those that need no outside agent — that would actually be helpful to a perfectly healthy existence? My answer is an unequivocal yes. Mental techniques exist that are far more enjoyable and life enhancing to practice than using alcohol, nicotine, and other toxic drugs. We will explore them in the second half of this book.

6

Weight Control and Obesity

OBESITY IS THE MOST COMMON metabolic disorder in affluent so-cieties. A person is said to be obese and not merely overweight when he reaches a level more than 10 percent above his ideal body weight. How is that determined? One simple way to approximate ideal body weight is as follows: For men of medium frame, the standard weight is calculated as 106 pounds for the first five feet of height and 6 pounds for each additional inch. One can add or subtract 10 percent of the result for large and small frames respectively. For women, the standard weight is 100 pounds for the first five feet of height and 5 pounds for each additional inch. Again, one can add or subtract 10 percent of this total for large and small frames respectively. Thus a man of medium frame, five feet eight inches tall, should weigh about 106 plus 48, or 154 pounds. A woman that tall should weigh 100 plus 40 pounds. Anyone who weighs more than 10 percent over this ideal body weight is consid-ered fat.

Obesity is not merely unattractive. It is in itself unhealthy and also predisposes a person to a number of illnesses. Being fat is def-initely linked to the following problems:

1. Heart conditions: Obesity places an increased burden on the heart and is known to be associated with enlargement of the heart. This can be reversed if the patient loses weight. Obesity is also linked to congestive heart failure and to coronary artery disease.

2. Joint deterioration: Because extra weight is added to the skeleton, obesity is linked to degenerative joint disease (osteoarthritis). Fat people are also more likely to suffer attacks of gouty arthritis. Attempting to lose weight with drastic high-protein fad diets can also cause attacks of gout.

3. Lung disturbance: Since extra body weight places a burden on the lungs by making breathing difficult, lung function is impaired. In particular, inadequate oxygen enters the blood because of labored breathing. This accounts for the fatigue that obese people complain of frequently.

4. Hypertension: Hardening of the arteries (atherosclerosis) occurs more frequently among fat people, and they are the most frequently prone to high blood pressure as a result. This highly dangerous condition, which can be reversed through weight loss, is linked to numerous other illnesses, including angina pectoris and sudden death from heart failure.

5. Gallstones: Fat people, especially women, develop gallstones more often than normal. Being overweight is associated with high levels of cholesterol secretion in the gallbladder, which leads to the formation of cholesterol gallstones.

6. Diabetes: About 80 percent of diabetics who develop this illness as adults are obese. Obesity adversely affects the fat cells so that they do not respond properly to insulin, and the result is elevated blood sugar, or diabetes. Many obese diabetics who are currently treated by medication, usually insulin injections, could be free of it simply by losing their excess weight.

7. Cancer: I have already talked about the great interest doctors are showing in the connection between diet and cancer. It appears that excessive eating in itself may stimulate production of the hormone estrogen, which is implicated in the onset of cancer. Also, obese women, particularly after menopause, are more prone

to cancer of the breast and uterus. Obesity is also a risk factor for prostate cancer in men.

This list could go on to include fatty liver illness, varicose veins, and high surgical risk whenever fat people need to be operated on for any reason. Fortunately, many of the potential health risks of being overweight disappear when the extra weight is dropped.

How does obesity occur? Very simply put, the body gains weight when the intake of calories exceeds what the body needs for physical activity and growth. Like almost every other physician, I see patients every day who come in wanting to lose weight. They consult me because they think they have a "gland problem." Most of them do not. They simply eat too much. Most of them have resorted to various diets and have lost weight, only to regain it over time. This is the familiar syndrome of losing and gaining the same five pounds every year. Because these people are frustrated and unhappy, they hope that a physician will diagnose some definite glandular disorder and relieve them of their malady. Some in fact do have a hormone or glandular disorder, such as underactive thyroid or tumor of the pituitary. In such cases a clear course of treatment emerges; therefore, I urge people who have been repeatedly unsuccessful at dieting to have a physical examination, which will disclose with laboratory tests the possibility of endocrine, hormonal, or metabolic problems.

The ordinary patient who simply eats too much would lose weight if he regularly followed a diet. The purpose of this book is not to recommend any commercial diet — some are clearly sensible and some are not. The basic principle behind all the sensible ones is that you must consume fewer calories than you expend if you intend to lose weight. All I need to add at this point is that for any diet to be permanently successful, you have to enjoy being on it. In fact, you should not feel that you are on a diet at all. Everyone should eat a weight-controlling and healthful diet, not because he thinks it is good for him and will make him lose weight, but because he would honestly prefer not to eat anything else.

So once again we are drawn to positive concepts like preference and enjoyment. They reflect attitudes that reside in the mind. I would like to emphasize that for most people being fat resides in the mind, and its cure will be in technologies that affect the mind and its basic outlook. Let me explain what I mean more specifically.

Very often one encounters the overweight person's complaint, "All I have to do is look at food and I gain weight." In many cases this may literally be true, according to experts who deal with obesity. They have shown that some people have a metabolic response to the sight or smell of food, or to the sound of cooking, which cannot be distinguished from the response they have when actually eating. In these people even the thought of food, working along a hormonal pathway from the pituitary to the adrenal gland to the pancreas, causes a rise of insulin in the blood stream. Insulin in turn causes irresistible hunger pangs and speeds up the process that converts food already eaten into fat. Experiments at Yale have also shown a dramatic rise in insulin levels when overweight patients are asked to watch the grilling of a thick, juicy steak.

Quite a few diet specialists now counsel their patients to avoid any situation that provokes these responses. These patients should routinely avoid glossy, attractive food ads and commercials on TV that glamorize food. They should not frequent restaurants or delis, even when they are going with a friend. In fact, ideally they should not dine with friends who have no weight problem, since they might be cajoled into eating by someone else's attitudes. Needless to say, they should not stand in front of bakery windows "just for a peek." Thoughts of food should be replaced, but without straining, by other pleasant images.

Another fascinating observation along these same lines, which many physicians would corroborate, is that drastic dieting can cause patients to *stop* losing weight altogether. It has even been noted, though the mechanism for this is not exactly known, that compared with moderate dieting, drastic dieting actually can lead to weight gain. One theory about this phenomenon holds that severe caloric restriction prompts the body to lower its rate of metabolic activity, so that although fewer calories are taken in, the body decides to burn fewer of them up. Instead, even these limited calories are turned into fat. It is as if the body sees a famine coming when so little food is eaten, so quite intelligently it decides to shut down its consumption and stores what little there is as future fuel.

Each body seems to have a set point that is a major determinant for its metabolic rate. This set point regulates the conversion of food either into energy or into muscles and fat. In effect it works like a thermostat, so that eating too much food or too little causes the metabolism to adjust in order to maintain a set balance; this is what makes it hard for people to change their "set" weight. But what determines the set point? It is difficult to say, but current information shows that self-image, a mental concept of how one looks, has a lot to do with it. A deeply held image of oneself as fat tends to keep that as the reality. The only effective therapy, then, is to try to change the set point through a change in mental self-image. Bringing the set point back to ideal body weight is after all what nature intends by setting up such a self-regulating mechanism, and many people who eat all they want but do not gain weight are simply obeying their inner sense of balance. What they want to eat and what their bodies want happen to agree.

Obese people may be suffering the consequences of a faulty body image. Everyone has an image of himself, but feeling fat or ugly or sickly interferes with the body's translation of the correct image into reality. Healthy people at ideal weight are projecting the attitude, "This is the body I was meant to have — it is healthy and beautiful." How can a healthy attitude of this kind be given to those who lack it? Neurophysiologists are evolving such techniques, working with the bodily mechanisms that connect self-image with the metabolic set point. I think that their approach is very important for treating obesity and a great many other conditions besides. When we think, "All I have to do is look at food and I gain weight," that becomes a reality because we are using (in a way we don't like) the psychophysiological connection. There is no reason why it should not also work in our favor.

7

Chronic Fatigue

FATIGUE OF ALL SORTS — weariness, listlessness, languor, depleted energy, loss of ambition, weakness — is one of the commonest symptoms patients bring to a doctor's office. The symptoms of fatigue can occur in a wide variety of medical settings, among them chronic infections, congestive heart failure, and debilitating illnesses such as cancer. People addicted to smoking, alcohol, or drugs experience fatigue when they begin to withdraw from their habit. In these situations, fatigue is not the primary medical problem. It accompanies a more primary condition and is often associated with a more distressing primary syndrome, such as shortness of breath.

Fatigue can be produced in any person through overwork and inadequate rest. The overwork does not have to be physical, either; chronically overworking oneself mentally, as well as physically, results in chronic fatigue. Anyone fatigued from overwork may not complain of fatigue as such. The problem may show itself instead through the symptoms of restlessness, insomnia, and irritability. Chronic fatigue can have deleterious effects on an otherwise healthy body. It can lead to the loss from muscle tissues of a complex carbohydrate called glycogen and the accumulation in the blood of toxic chemicals such as lactic acid. Interestingly, researchers have found that injecting blood from a fatigued animal into a rested animal produces in it all the signs of fatigue. This suggests that the symptoms of fatigue come about through the action of toxins that have been released into the blood stream by muscles and other organs.

Enough clinical evidence exists to indicate that fatigue changes the metabolism of the affected person. Fatigued patients often display a faster breath rate, faster pulse, dilated pupils, and higher blood pressure. Their blood count may show an increase in the number of white cells. All of these physiological signs are exactly the opposite of those seen in a person who is deeply resting through sleep or through the restful but alert state of meditation. Even though the physiology appears speeded up after overwork, fatigue obviously does not enhance activity. People afflicted with chronic fatigue cannot work as much or as well; they feel an inability to deal with life's common problems or to make correct decisions. This inability to judge situations realistically leads to common signs of irrational behavior and irritability.

When fatigue is a secondary symptom associated with a primary disease condition, it is not difficult to manage since treatment consists of treating the disorder. The problem of treatment arises when fatigue is the primary complaint and investigation cannot uncover an illness to account for it. In these instances, the doctor usually will find other signs, such as nervousness, depression, loss of appetite and sexual drive, headaches, insomnia, irritability, and inability to concentrate. Patients with such complaints who are admitted to a hospital for "exhaustion" are in the vast number of instances eventually diagnosed as having either anxiety neurosis or depression. In one study, fully 75 percent of such patients were diagnosed as neurotically anxious, 10 percent as depressed, and the rest as suffering from a wide variety of psychological and physical disorders.

Several theories have been put forward to explain the development of fatigue in otherwise healthy people. Strong emotions like anxiety can trigger the release of chemicals into the blood stream (for example, cortisol and adrenaline) which in turn could lead to the accumulation of toxins. These toxins in the blood would then cause the outward manifestations of fatigue. So-called stage fright, a consequence of intense worry and anxiety, is one example of such a phenomenon. The strong emotion results in a sense of physical weakness, inability to act, confusion, and finally exhaustion.

This theory accounts for the enervation brought on by powerful emotions, but it does not explain the fatigue that appears without accompanying emotional episodes. Some psychologists have suggested that fatigue appears as a warning signal and that the symptoms of it are self-protecting. When some particular attitude or activity becomes too intense or too persistent, and therefore must be changed, the symptoms of fatigue show up as a means of self-preservation. They carry the message that something deeper is wrong. Some psychologists theorize that we carry within ourselves a host of unacceptable attitudes and ideas. We repress these ideas, that is, we keep them under wraps, and this effort requires the expenditure of mental force, which psychologists often call "psychic energy." When the strain of repression becomes great enough actually to deplete our store of psychic energy, then the physical signs of fatigue show up. Other psychologists have said that fatigue is not a self-protective mechanism but that it still comes from the unconscious, in this case from an unconscious wish to be inactive, for whatever hidden reason.

Despite these elegant and sometimes quite contradictory theories, some observations about fatigue are quite commonplace. Fatigue appears to be more usual among people who have no definite purpose in life. It appears among people who have too much time on their hands, who are bored or stuck in the monotony of daily routines. When these people find an opportunity to get out of their rut and take on new projects with a definite goal in mind, they commonly snap out of their fatigue automatically. They are overtaken by optimism and enthusiasm, and the memory that they were ever fatigued does not even crop up in their minds.

So fatigue may very well belong in the category of attitude problems. In my experience with patients, fatigue's most common causes are boredom, lack of curiosity, and an absence of enthusiasm. These causes represent definite states of mind, and their opposites are just as definite. Curiosity, enthusiasm, and eagerness for life are normal aspects of perfect health. We will come to them as we learn more about health as a state that we can create.

8

Gastrointestinal Disorders

DISORDERS OF THE STOMACH and intestines are very common and are sensitively connected to everyday situations. Anyone who has experienced butterflies or knots in the stomach during episodes of stress does not need to be convinced that the nervous system and the digestive system are intimately related. Biologically, the gastrointestinal system of the human embryo develops as an outgrowth of the nervous system. In an adult, the entire intestinal tract is abundantly supplied with nerves through the autonomic nervous system, the part of the nervous system that is automatically self-regulating. Also, a number of hormones in the gastrointestinal system have also been discovered to be present in the nervous system (for example, gastrin, secretin, glucagon, somatostain, and half a dozen more). The exact role these hormones play in the nervous system has yet to be defined.

It is sufficient to say that this connection between the neuroendocrine and digestive systems is there and will have important ramifications to researchers. This connection should further clarify a common observation, well known to all physicians, that many digestive problems are psychosomatic in character. In other words, attitudes of mind can show up in the digestive system as ulcers, irritable bowels, and various degrees of colitis, or inflamed colon. Because emotional problems at the very least serve to aggravate these common complaints, people who have ulcers or bowel difficulties frequently can look forward to no cure as long as their emotions are disturbed in daily life. Their symptoms may be relieved if they follow bland diets and take relaxants, antacids, and other drugs, but even when surgery is performed to remove damaged portions of the digestive tract, the chance that symptoms will reappear may last for years, even a lifetime.

Ulcers

The activity of stomach juices is strongly affected by the emotions. Ordinarily the lining of the stomach wall is protected from the powerful chemicals in the stomach, such as hydrochloric acid, but when this natural defense breaks down, the stomach literally starts to digest part of itself. An open sore then develops that is very slow to heal, and this is called a peptic ulcer. Ulcers frequently occur during periods of stress. People recognized as having "ulcer personalities," usually men, are hard driving, hurried, stubborn, critical, obstinate, worrisome, and emotional. Frequently they are also smokers and heavy drinkers as well and have bad dietary habits. Because they eat themselves up with work, it is no wonder that such people have stomachs that decide to do much the same thing.

Other factors enter into the cause of ulcers, such as a family history of ulcers or having type O blood, and the exact causes are still debated. Mild ulcers are treatable with a combination of a bland diet containing milk, antacids to neutralize stomach acids, and abstinence from alcohol, smoking, and caffeine. However, ulcers tend to recur despite these measures, and if untreated, the open sore may break all the way through the stomach lining (this is called perforation) resulting in the patient's death. No definite preventive is known, which means that ulcer victims may spend a lifetime watching their diet and strictly avoiding alcohol, caffeine, and cigarettes.

It is often quite difficult for people with "ulcer personalities" to do that, however. Since they watch themselves with a critical eye all the time, asking them to watch even more closely only makes them worse. Sometimes giving up alcohol and cigarettes, their only means of release, provokes so much tension for these people that their ulcers actually respond to treatment more poorly. Ulcers also tend to flair up during periods of emotional upset in people who are prone to this problem, regardless of how careful they have been.

Irritable Colon

Irritable colon syndrome is the most common gastrointestinal disorder seen in clinical practice. It causes considerable distress to patients and is extremely difficult to treat. The symptoms are lower abdominal pain with alternating constipation and diarrhea. Patients suffering from an irritable colon are known to have markedly increased life stress and mild neurotic personality traits. Specialists still debate whether these people are emotionally distressed because of their symptoms or whether the symptoms first appeared as a result of emotional disturbance — the two seem to go around in a vicious circle. The physical symptoms themselves are quite difficult to treat directly, but significantly, successfully treating the patient's neurotic symptoms usually causes the physical symptoms to disappear. And the successful treatment of the colon problems, particularly in milder cases, means that the immediate anxiety and worry also go away.

These are just further examples of what medicine is discovering when any disease process in any system is studied: it is the phenomenon of psyche affecting soma, mind affecting body. When a state of mind expresses itself in harmful changes of the physiology, the result is what we call a disease process.

9

Sexual Inadequacy

INCREASING NUMBERS of patients are willing to consult their physicians about sexual problems. In part this reflects a greater openness to discuss a topic that once was considered taboo, but in my view it also reflects a higher incidence of sexual dysfunction in the present generation. Society may be paying more attention to sex in the superficial context of journalism and entertainment, but that in part may be because people are more worried about it and more uncertain about what is normal and healthy. Sexual dysfunctions have classically fallen into two broad categories: changes of libido (sexual drive) or changes in the ability to perform and gain satisfaction. So far as daily medical practice is concerned, the most common complaints from women are failure to be aroused during love making and failure to achieve orgasm. In men the most frequent complaints are premature ejaculation and impotence.

Sexual Problems

Sexual Inadequacy in Women

Although in my opinion no really convincing ideas exist about the causes of sexual dysfunction in women, a number of factors appear to contribute. If a child senses that her parents, particularly the mother, have a negative attitude toward sex, or if a child who is innocent of sexual matters is traumatically exposed to a sexual encounter, then the adult woman may well develop sexual problems later. Another extremely common cause is that the woman may hold negative feelings, not necessarily sexual ones, toward her husband or partner, or toward marriage. Frequently she finds something in her husband's behavior that makes her consistently angry at him, though she may not openly show it. Or she may have had injunctions condemning sex deeply instilled in her by her parents or by religious instructors. Any of these can produce inhibitions that block sexual enjoyment.

Whatever the cause of the dysfunction, leaving aside an actual medical disorder that can be diagnosed and treated, the end result has a common feature: the patient begins to focus her mind on evaluating her performance and the state of her arousal. She cannot simply enjoy the act of sexual intercourse. Evaluative thoughts clearly inhibit the first relaxed stages of the human sexual response. Orgasm cannot be reached and allowed to take its own course because there is no enjoyment of the sexual setting in the first place. Orgasm is, after all, a peak experience, and it is only possible when it is experienced freely, without judgmental thoughts, for ideally, all thoughts are transcended in the moment. Almost every study of this problem has concluded that anxious overconcern about performance contributes to sexual inadequacy in women.

Sexual Inadequacy in Men

Premature ejaculation, which has been defined as ejaculating before either one or both partners desire it, is entirely a psychological problem. Whether it is classified as a reflex or as a learned response that has hidden motivations behind it, this most common of male sexual complaints exists in the mind. Masters and Johnson concluded from their research that premature ejaculation was learned during a man's first sexual encounters, which he associated with guilt, time pressure, or fear of being detected.

Impotence is the inability to obtain or sustain an erection when there is sexual desire for it. This condition does have some medical causes, among them hormonal disorders of the pituitary, thyroid, or testes. It also can appear in diabetics or in anyone weakened from illness or suffering the side effects of debilitating drug treatments. Alcohol and marijuana, among other drugs, can also induce episodes of impotence, particularly among heavy users. In the majority of patients, however, this too is a psychological problem. Fears or guilt associated with sex or anxiety about performance are often responsible. Of these, a fixed preoccupation with performance seems to be the most important factor. It masks a fear of failure that is making natural arousal impossible.

Loss of Libido

In both sexes, the decrease of desire for sex, or loss of libido, usually has an emotional or other psychological cause lying behind it. However, it is also common to see loss of sex drive when alcohol, opiates, and marijuana are used. People may casually assume that drugs increase libido and add to sexual potency, but this is not the case. Drugs can increase sexual *activity* by removing inhibitions, but the activity is inadequate for the most part because these drugs have a depressive effect on the central nervous system. Because they "provoke the desire, but take away the performance," to paraphrase Shakespeare, alcohol and drugs do not lend themselves to healthy sexual enjoyment. As for the psychological causes of lessened sexual desire, depression appears to be the most common, but fear, insecurity, and guilt can also be responsible.

Approaches to Treating Sexual Disorders

I believe that successful approaches to treating sexual inadequacy revolve around changing the patient's thought patterns. Sex is a wonderful and beautiful part of our lives. Like all other basic instincts, it has its origin in the mind. The attitude of mind that permits it to flow is open, undemanding, and innocent. The thought patterns that favor a spontaneous enjoyment of sex exist in people who can also be loving and giving. It is a mistake to think that the amount of sex in one's life is crucial, that more is better. Sexual activity is good only when its enemies are absent, and they are fear, frustration, and repression.

The modern clinical approach to treating sexual problems generally focuses on changing unsuccessful behavior. A common technique is known as "systematic desensitization." Essentially this approach looks on sexual inadequacy as a product of faulty learning in which sex is associated with fear and tension. The aim, then, is to relearn about sex and eliminate sexual fears in a step-by-step process. The patient is taken through stages of voluntary muscle relaxation, then he lists sexual situations in the order of increasing anxiety that they pose for him, and finally he exposes these situations to the relaxation technique by visualizing them and learning to relax at the same time. Other styles of behavior modification deal with sexual situations physically, but all are attempting to remove the fears that have been ingrained by faulty early training.

These approaches have clearly proved useful, particularly for treating impotence and failure of orgasm, but sexual inadequacy remains a widespread problem. I think it is one because there has been too much concern and deliberate cerebration about something that is natural, instinctive, and spontaneous. When people are enjoying a state of perfect health, there are no sexual problems. Instead of worrying about how much or how good, healthy people put sex back into its proper place as a private part of their lives that they express through love of another person.

When patients ask for sexual counseling, I take advantage of the fact that sex is one of the most powerful and spontaneous of natural urges. I tell them to leave it alone. When left alone and not dwelt upon, sex begins to stir. Men do not achieve erection by willing it, but that is just what a worried, preoccupied man will try to do. It comes as a relief when the doctor tells him that he is forbidden to think about sex or to try to engage in it. These patients who were totally preoccupied with sex and unable to enjoy it now find that enjoyment and spontaneity return just because they try so hard not even to entertain sex as a possibility. By turning their attention to "leaving it alone," I am simply allowing them to remove the obstacles that interfere with spontaneity. The change that takes place happens, once again, at the level of the mind where health wants to assert itself as an irresistible force.

10

Sleep and Insomnia

SLEEP IS ENTIRELY NATURAL, absolutely necessary, and yet mostly still a mystery. Only recently have even the basic facts about sleep been researched, and why it is needed or how it works to restore us in mind and body has yet to be discovered. It is known that men and women do not differ in the hours they sleep. Most people, about 60 percent, sleep between six and eight hours a night, about 36 percent sleep more than eight hours, and below 4 percent less than six hours. No one has ever been found not to sleep at all, and very few people can successfully change the time that they naturally sleep by conscious effort. In a study of thousands of people, about 57 percent of both men and women reported that they wake up feeling refreshed after a night's sleep, leaving a great many who do not. Of those who suffer from insomnia, the ratio of men to women show its first significant difference: women outnumber men about two to one in reporting that they have spent at least one totally sleepless night. Women also take sleeping aids more often than men in about this same proportion.

Physiologists have discovered two general kinds of sleep in mammals, including humans. These are rapid eye movement, or REM, sleep and slow wave, or non-REM, sleep. Within these categories, however, there are many levels of light and heavy, unconscious and semiconscious sleep. REM sleep has attracted much research and public attention because it is the sleep phase in which dreams occur. It is believed that this phase is responsible for the rest and rejuvenation we derive from sleep.

As is now commonly known, we need both to sleep and to dream in order to feel restored in the morning. Although many people, especially chronic insomniacs, claim to be completely sleepless or completely without dreams, in fact this belief exists only in their minds. To go without sleeping and dreaming quickly creates severely abnormal brain functioning.

Our pattern of alternating rest and activity in a cycle links us with all living species. In fact, REM sleep has been found in birds, reptiles, and fish and is a distinctive mark of where a species belongs on the ladder of evolution. As I will discuss in more detail later on, functions like sleep show that our nervous system is interconnected with all the primary vital qualities of nature. Our ordinary cycle of sleeping, dreaming, and waking binds us with all things in the universe.

The pattern of sleep in human beings varies during different periods of life. Sleeping mostly at night appears as early as the first few weeks of life and continues into old age. Then, however, the pattern begins to break down. Old people generally report not only that they sleep less — sometimes five or six hours of sleep a night is normal for them — but also that they exhibit a new sleep pattern of waking in the night and napping during the day.

Researchers looking into the unanswered question of how sleep works have theorized that daily fatigue produces a substance in us called a hypnotoxin which activates a portion of the brain, the reticular formation, to bring on the sleep response. Sleep is not only a state of consciousness, it is also a state of altered body chemistry. If spinal fluid is taken from a sleeping cat, for instance, and injected into the spine of a cat that is wide awake, that cat will fall asleep immediately. In the same way, we wake up when the brain secretes the necessary chemicals to counteract the ones that keep us asleep. Allowing these biological processes to take place normally and according to our own personal sleep rhythms is an important part of a healthy life.

Sleep deprivation quickly leads to a loss of well-being. If experimental animals are deprived of sleep for even a few days, they die. In humans, sleep deprivation begins by causing fatigue, irritability, and loss of concentration. It soon leads, however, to physical and mental disorientation, to delusions and hallucinations, and to a progressive decline in the ability to perform any coordinated movements at all. Later stages are intensely uncomfortable because they induce the symptoms of actual neurological disease, including muscle weakness, defective vision, and slurred speech.

Apparently about a quarter of adult Americans need drugs to sleep, to judge by the sale of sleeping aids. In treating insomnia, physicians write prescriptions for hypnotics and sedatives, a class of drugs that accounts for more prescriptions than any other. In its most common variety, insomnia is not related to any physical disorder. It can occur in connection with pain, certain organic illnesses, and drug use, but the usual causes of insomnia are nervousness, worry, and anxiety. Insomnia frequently accompanies more serious psychological problems (for example manic depression or depression by itself), and in these conditions both the quantity and quality of sleep are seriously impaired. By poor quality, we mean that all the stages of the sleep cycle are not fully experienced, particularly REM sleep. One characteristic of depression is early morning awakening, where the patient has no difficulty falling asleep but then wakes up at 2:00 or 3:00 A.M. and cannot fall asleep again. Many anxious people also find that they wake up very suddenly, almost with a "click," and are immediately aware of their racing, nervous thoughts.

The research investigating the biochemistry and brain functioning of sleep has also been directed at finding sleep-producing drugs. These range from simple, relatively inert compounds sold over the counter to more effective (and habit-forming) drugs like barbiturates and a new class of drugs called benzodiazepines. All drugs prescribed for insomnia share a characteristic drawback, and that is drug tolerance — after a short period of use they are no longer effective. Patients who regularly need sleeping pills require larger and larger doses to get the same effect. These drugs also do not provide the right quality of sleep because they interfere with periods of REM sleep. The stupor induced by too much alcohol may resemble sleep, but it too deprives one of REM sleep. The poor quality of drug-produced sleep is attested to by the patients when they complain of morning hangovers, fatigue, constipation, loss of energy and sexual drive, and an inability to recover quickly from illness. When these drugs are withdrawn, some patients experience delirium and hallucination. It seems clear, then, that research aimed at finding a pharmaceutical solution to sleeplessness is misdirected.

It takes no more than common sense to realize that when we cannot fall asleep, it is our thoughts that keep us awake. Worry and anxiety are nothing but negative thoughts about something that has already occurred or about something that might occur in the future (but usually does not). Sometimes, of course, it is a happy thought, an anticipation of some happy occurrence that keeps us awake. We usually do not mind that sort of sleeplessness, however, since any sleep that does eventually come is ordinarily quite refreshing. Good health in general is indicated by restful sleep, and the quality of sleep one is used to indicates the state of mental and physical well-being that one is also used to. Happy, contented, loving people seldom suffer from insomnia. People ridden with guilt, anxiety, and unhappiness suffer it routinely. One does not need the support of science to verify this fact, which people have known throughout the ages. Sleep disorders are practically unknown among children (unless there is present a severely painful illness or an actual mental disturbance).

Children can sleep well because they are innocent. If we expect to approach adult sleep disorders successfully, we will need to begin with the thought patterns that are not innocent, that interfere with what should be completely automatic and free of preoccupation. Deep within the mind, at the source of thought, we will find our answers.

11

Stress and the Burned-out Syndrome

MEDICAL RESEARCHERS have been suspicious of stress for quite a long time, but in the last decade it became obvious that stress is indeed a major cause of disease and even death. It is implicated now in almost every disease from heart disorders and hypertension to cancer, not leaving out diabetes, assorted metabolic problems, and hormonal disorders such as diseased thyroid.

What exactly is stress? Dr. Hans Selye is credited with first using the word as it applies to the physiology, and he defined it as the nonspecific response of the body to any demand made upon it. He described a "general adaptation syndrome" in which the body reacts to any threatening stimulus through a predictable sequence of internal changes, including the release of certain hormones. This is familiar to all of us as the fight-or-flight response that occurs when we are physically endangered. As the term implies, these responses evolved in us, and in all living things, as a protective mechanism. They are what enables all organisms to respond to changes in their environment. Although Selye thought that one predictable series of responses arose in the face of all stressors, whether they were physical or psychological, it now appears that this is not really the case.

Scientists now believe that organisms possess quite individualized and specific responses to outside threats. The standard definition of stress now more closely fits what people ordinarily think of when they apply the term to themselves: "Stress is the accumulation of normal and abnormal pressures of daily living that test the individual's ability to cope." Anyone who spends his energies coping with the speed, noise, and chaos of things as they are today can identify with this definition.

However, it is commonly assumed that stress is something outside ourselves, that it *is* the speed, noise, and chaos. This view is in error; stress is inside us. According to Dr. Daniel X. Friedman, an authority on stress, "Stress is a coupled action of the *body and mind* involving *appraisal* of a threat, an instant modulation of response. The triggering mechanism is the individual's *perception* of threat, not an event. Perception is modified by temperament and experience." The italics are mine, added to point to the subjective nature of stress. Dr. Friedman goes on to say that everyone responds to outer threats in his own way, depending on "previous level of arousal and ability to adapt. Appropriate stress helps the individual to adapt. Inappropriate stress, however, serves no useful purpose and may result in disease."

So it is the individual's perception of threat and not the event itself that triggers stress. This is very important for us to see. Let us take a few examples. The most frequently cited stressors, or sources of stress, in our lives include divorce, death of a loved one, loss of money, possessions, or a job, disease in a close relative, and criticism from other people. However, these are not the real stressors. The real stressors are fear of divorce, fear of losing a loved one, fear of losing a job, and fear of criticism. Even imminent death in itself is not so much the threat as one's fear of dying. Once again we come back to ideas, to brain patterns that excite biochemical and neural changes. The stress is acting along these pathways from mind to body.

Considerable research data now exist to tell us about the hormonal and related biochemical changes that take place under stressful conditions. Cortisol, a hormone secreted by the adrenal glands, rises in response to a wide variety of stressful events. Many reports, for instance, showed that cortisol increases when people have to undergo surgery. More detailed study of these reports, however, revealed that it was not the surgery itself, but the *anticipation* of surgery that caused the rise in cortisol levels. Another hormone studied under stressful conditions was the growth hormone. It was shown to be elevated in students when they took exams or when they were asked to view violent or sexually explicit scenes from movies. Significantly, it also rose if students *anticipated* exhausting exercise or were faced with tests that provoke distress and anxiety.

Other hormones whose levels rise in similar circumstances include epinephrine, norepinephrine, and prolactin, a pituitary hormone. All of these examples prove that stress operates through the psychophysiological connection: a thought results in the secretion of a hormone, usually a group of hormones, that in turn leads to many changes in the body's metabolism and physiology. To put it in simple and very general terms, a person perceives a threat, his brain registers the threat by sending out signals to trigger the release of hormones, and the hormones serve as messengers to the parts of the body that need to react. And this stress response, which can throw the whole body into powerful action, takes place in only a few thousandths of a second.

How does the stress response manifest itself in abnormal ways? Often it manifests itself as a disease. Since disease involves a great many changes over time, we should say that stress shows up as a disease *process* whose effects accumulate in the body. The process can result in hypertension in one person and ulcers in another (there is a saying in medicine, "Ulcers are not what you eat, but what is eating you"). Or stress may manifest itself in nonspecific symptoms of the kind that constitute what is commonly referred to as "burned-out syndrome."

What people experience when they "burn out," and what doctors are increasingly recognizing, is exhaustion on all levels of body, emotions, and life attitudes.. The physical complaints include fatigue, insomnia, headaches, backaches, bad digestion, shortness of breath, lingering colds, and undesired weight loss or gain. The emotions and attitude toward life are likely to change in the direction of boredom, restlessness, a feeling of stagnation, and depression. Burned-out people get through the day by rationalizing their behavior or indulging in obsessive activities and thoughts. Compared with people in the healthy state of welcoming life, the burned-out show quick irritation, cannot compliment other people or enjoy their successes, and react to daily events with cynicism, defensiveness, and fault finding. In order to gain some release from themselves they frequently become dependent on alcohol or drugs.

The stress response may also prove to be lethal. A striking recent discovery about stress is that it depletes the immune system of the body. When a person is under chronic stress, production of the body's natural "killer" cells, called T-lymphocytes and macrophages, seems to be inhibited. Perhaps this inhibition occurs because of the excessive levels of cortisol and other hormones that are observed in stressed people. Since these killer cells are responsible for fighting against infections and other disease, we may have found the link that connects stress and the development of disorders like pneumonia and cancer.

Is stress necessary in some way? Sometimes stressed people rationalize their unhealthy state by declaring that they need stress in order to perform well, by which they usually mean that they need stress in order to compete and be successful in their rushed existences. Articles have appeared stating much the same thing, that some stress is good for you but too much, particularly too much of the wrong kind, is bad. I think this attitude is utterly wrong. All living organisms have innate mechanisms that allow them to grow and adapt. The sunflower follows the sun across the sky because an inner mechanism controls that behavior, and on cloudy days the mechanism quite automatically shows the intelligence not to operate. What we see here is that adaptations are appropriate and natural. Human beings are endowed with the widest and most creative range of such mechanisms in all of nature. Our ability to adapt has no end to it. In a perfectly healthy person, the natural, appropriate response is at hand for every situation. This includes the response of not doing anything, of showing patience and silence, and of knowing when to rest.

However, when we strain to react unnaturally, to interfere with the responses that already reside in our intelligence, then problems begin. Stress accumulates when we do not live according to our inner intelligence. To say that we need *more* stress in the form of more aroused behavior is like saying that we need to learn to adjust to the abnormalities of strain, overcompetition, and constant hurrying. This argument obviously shows a great distrust of the body's inner intelligence. "Stress management" can only be successful when there is no management. An infinite variety of responses already guides us through life and given the chance will never fail to meet the situations of living. However, these responses have to be instantaneously coordinated if they are to work as nature intended. The mind can make decisions, but so can the heart, so can the hormonal pathways, so can each cell, and so can the DNA at the center of each cell. When they all act in harmony, the result is perfect health and natural, life-enhancing intelligence. All we need in order to take full advantage of this is a life that is without strain, and for that a trusting, relaxed attitude is most important.

Such are the myriad manifestations of the stress response. The key to all of them lies in the one place that this book is all about — the human mind, the origin of all thoughts and of all bodily processes that begin with thoughts. We will discover that much of the current controversy about stress and how to manage it becomes pointless once we aim our therapies at the deepest level of health.

Instead of the medical definitions of stress, I prefer one expressed by Maharishi Mahesh Yogi, an authority on consciousness from the Eastern perspective: "Stress is that which blocks the full expression of creative intelligence." Given this definition, a person without stress becomes a model of life, a human being living to the full potential of his intelligence.

12

Emotional Illness and Depression

A MAJOR CONTROVERSY has arisen in medicine over the origin of emotional disorders and particularly depression, which afflicts millions of people. During an attack of depression a person feels sad and drained, without the ability to enjoy life or to overcome the general feeling of fatigue and weakness that in serious cases is practically paralyzing. There is also usually an accompanying feeling of anxiety, loss of appetite, and insomnia. No one clearly understands why such attacks occur, and in those seriously prone to depression, bouts of it become longer and more frequent over time, until eventually they see no reason to live. The present debate has to do with whether such people should be treated psychiatrically, which means with counseling, or medically, which means with drugs. The recent publicity given to successful treatment with chemical antidepressants has made the public aware that not only depression, but all sorts of disorders "in the head" also have consequences in the body as well.

We now can confidently say that a wide variety of psychological disorders are associated not just with mental symptoms, but with definite biochemical profiles:

Major depression: A number of biochemical disturbances can be seen in patients suffering from depression. In fact, it will soon become commonplace for physicians to run blood tests to aid in diagnosing this disorder. Among the most notable changes are increased secretion of the hormone cortisol from the adrenal glands, deficient secretion of the growth hormone, deficient secretion of the thyroid-stimulating hormone (TSH), and elevated levels of prolactin, which is secreted by the pituitary.

Schizophrenia: This is a serious psychological disorder in young adults. More than a million people suffer from it in this country, though precisely what it is has not been agreed upon. Schizophrenics lose touch with reality and suffer from many severe symptoms, such as delusion, hallucinations, and disordered thinking. An acute attack of schizophrenia renders the person incapable of functioning in society, and in the past this required putting the patient in an asylum because of his excitement, agitation, restlessness, and irrational behavior. This is now the other major psychological disorder besides depression (and a variation called manic depression) that can be routinely treated with drugs. People with this disease display abnormalities in several pituitary hormones, including the growth hormone, gonadotropins, which are the sex hormones, and prolactin. Other brain and endocrine hormones may also be involved, however.

Anorexia nervosa: This is an eating disorder, now widely publicized, that mainly affects young women and adolescent girls. The patient is morbidly afraid of gaining weight and imagines her body to be fatter than in reality it is. This idea persists even when the body has nearly been starved to death. Anorectics reject food in order to continue to lose weight. Sometimes the disorder alternates with bulimia, uncontrolled binge eating that is followed by remorse and shame (the bingeing is dealt with by inducing vomiting in secret), or the two disorders can exist separately. The biochemical profile of anorexia also shows abnormal pituitary secretions involving the growth hormone, as well as sex hormones such as the follicle-stimulating hormone and the luteinizing hormone.

All of these disorders (and the list could be considerably lengthened) are very stubborn when treated psychiatrically, but this does not mean that chemical cures have been found. Drugs for treating the mind, even when relatively successful, always have side effects. Some of the drugs used to calm the disordered thought processes in schizophrenics are broad and drastic in reducing normal thought in these patients as well — they are sometimes called "chemical straitjackets." The revolution in treating mental disturbance with drugs has brought relief to some people and has emptied beds in mental hospitals, but no one can claim that a majority of these patients has been healed.

One can make the simple observation that in mental illness disturbing thought patterns cause biochemical changes in the body. The controversy over which came first, the emotional disturbance or the chemical change, to me seems irrelevant. It doesn't matter which came first so long as we observe, in the words of the old riddle, that chickens do come from eggs and eggs from chickens.

To give an example, there is an uncommon disorder known as psychosocial dwarfism in which children display delayed puberty and markedly reduced size (about 50 percent of the normal height for their age group), as well as retarded bone age. These children usually come from emotionally deprived families. Tests of their blood show a much lower level of growth hormone than is normal. When these children are removed to an emotionally supportive environment, however, they rapidly begin to grow and even tend to catch up with their age norms. Importantly, when they start to improve clinically, the level of growth hormone in their blood is also seen to increase at the same time. Other children with the "maternal deprivation syndrome" exhibit the apathetic and withdrawn behavior that was deeply ingrained in them by an early lack of warm, close mothering. These children withdraw from social contact and even appear insensitive to physical pain; they often inflict injury on themselves. At intervals outbursts of temper and disruptiveness appear. Yet once again, if they are treated in an emotionally warm environment by loving, caring, and compassionate people, the biochemical abnormalities that "cause" their abnormal behavior are seen to reverse.

In other words, the body chemistry of these children has responded in one way to the emotions of fear, anxiety, and depression but in quite another way to love and compassion. What we are seeing here is that there is no real duality, no *real* psychophysiological connection. We create the connection — meaning that we have divided mind and body in the first place — so that we can understand the physiology. In the field of the psyche, Sigmund Freud made his breakthrough in psychology by seeing that there is no *real* duality between the thoughts of disturbed people and so-called normal thought; rather, all thinking takes place on a line that runs continuously through human experience. Now we can extend the line to include the physiology, which is ultimately an expression of the same unified organism that we call human. At a subtle level, this organism is just an expression of thought processes and excitations of intelligence in the field of "mind." That is the view we are leading up to when we examine the mind-body connection.

The implications of this for mental therapy are very significant, I think. People who suffer from depression or other psychological maladies are victims of shattered wholeness. Once they step out of the state in which mind and body are healthy together, then dozens and dozens of symptoms, mental and physical, can burden them. We say that some are mental and others are physiological. Depending on the physician's viewpoint, the treatment for them may be through psychiatry or through drugs. But essentially a single thing — wholeness of mind and body — has been lost. It is beyond our powers to restore this wholeness by trying to alleviate every symptom. Wholeness must be restored from within — that must be obvious by now — and this process begins only when we grasp the subtlest level of the human organism, the "self."

13

The Psychophysiological Connection — Some Dramatic Case Histories

WE HAVE NOW SEEN that the psychophysiological connection plays a crucial role in the onset of disease processes. It is just as important in their outcome. Patients are drastically different in the way their minds and bodies react to illness. The following case histories reveal some dramatic instances of that.

Case No. 1

A forty-two-year-old business executive named Mr. Avery* phoned me to say he had been having mild intermittent chest pains for several months. His description of the pain was suggestive of angina pectoris, which results when there is decreased blood supply to the heart. He said that the pain came on when he was depressed, anxious, or hurriedly trying to make a deadline at

* I have changed the names and concealed the identities of people described in these case histories.

work. The pain did not occur when he exercised. This description suggested that his pain was due to spasm of the coronary vessels, the arteries feeding blood to the heart, as opposed to a fixed narrowing of these vessels which occurs in hardening of the arteries. I advised him to come to the office for a checkup. At that, he got extremely upset, saying that he had no time and that there was "no way" he could leave his business projects, even for a minute.

However, the episodes of pain increased in frequency, and he finally had to agree to an office visit. He became extremely agitated in the waiting room because he had to wait for fifteen minutes, and he began to shout at my receptionist, declaring that he was an extremely busy man who had no time to waste and that I should not have made an appointment for him if I could not see him immediately. When I saw him in the examining room shortly thereafter, he was extremely angry — he started off by telling me that doctors thought only their time was valuable and that they had no regard for the patient's time. After examining him, I informed him that he was probably having attacks of unstable angina pectoris. In my opinion, he should be admitted to the hospital for further diagnostic tests.

When Mr. Avery heard this, he lost control of himself. He ranted and raved about the impossibility of taking my advice. I could see that he was beginning to froth around the mouth and was losing color from his face. At that moment, he clutched at his chest and fell to the floor. It was obvious that he had suffered a cardiac arrest, and I attempted resuscitative measures, but to no avail. Twenty minutes after this patient walked into my office, he was dead. The autopsy later revealed what we had suspected: the patient had suffered a myocardial infarct, a heart attack. But the autopsy also revealed that his coronary arteries were clean; there was no obstruction of the sort seen when an artery is clogged. The heart attack had been caused instead by spasm of the coronary vessels, directly induced by hostility, resentment, impatience, fear, and exaggerated feelings of being indispensable.

Mr. Avery had been killed in a matter of two minutes by his

thoughts. I have detailed the mechanism behind this phenomenon already, but basically powerful negative emotions, thoughts of hostility and fear, induce complex physiological changes through the release of hormones via the pituitary-adrenal axis. The wave of change in the body is dramatic, rapid, and complicated to unravel, but we can determine that blood pressure rises, as does heartbeat, and even the coronary vessels can go into spasm, as occurred here.

Case No. 2

I was asked to see a forty-six-year-old foreign patient named Mr. Patel who had been admitted to the coronary care unit of a local teaching hospital in the Boston area. He was visiting Boston from India and had been attending business conferences when he suffered a heart attack. In the intensive care unit of the hospital he developed life-threatening arrhythmias, that is, abnormal heart rhythms of the kind that impair contraction and therefore make it difficult for the heart to pump blood effectively.

This patient had suffered the most serious kind of arrhythmia, called ventricular fibrillation. In ventricular fibrillation the heartbeat is virtually ineffective; it is a kind of rapid fluttering. This can often follow a heart attack and is caused by electrical instability in the heart. Unless the patient is immediately resuscitated, usually by applying electric shock to the chest, death rapidly ensues. Mr. Patel had already gone through several episodes of fibrillating and fortunately had been brought back each time with electric shock. It was not clear why he kept going into these spurts of arrhythmia. It was clear, however, that if these episodes continued for much longer, he would not leave the hospital alive.

When I saw him, I found out that he was extremely worried about how he was going to pay his bill. Because he was visiting from another country, he was not covered by hospital insurance, and he had heard from other people that "in America, if you are hospitalized without medical insurance, you will live in debt for the rest of your life." He told me that he would rather die than spend the rest of his years in debt. I reassured him by telling him that his bill would be taken care of, despite what he had heard, and that in fact, unbeknownst to him, his company had taken out a special travel policy for him and his entire delegation. After he was given this news, his vital signs stabilized, and he had no further episodes of ventricular fibrillation. He was discharged in three weeks and left the country for home a week later, completely free of symptoms. Had they not been allayed in time, this patient's fearful thoughts would almost certainly have killed him. I never did find out who paid his hospital bill.

Case No. 3

Mr. Badgett, a thirty-five-year-old lawyer, came to the emergency room of the hospital complaining of nonspecific chest pain. After a careful examination, the emergency room doctor assured him that everything was all right; the chest pain was muscular in origin. The patient no sooner reached home than the chest pain recurred, and he returned to the emergency room. This time I was asked to examine him. After giving him a thorough physical and examining his electrocardiogram (EKG), which was normal, I decided to admit him for observation nevertheless because of his severe anxiety. Twenty-four hours later, I found that there were indeed some changes in his EKG which suggested that he had suffered some damage to his heart. These changes had not initially been apparent when Mr. Badgett came to the emergency room.

When I told him about this, the patient turned quite upset and angry. He immediately informed me that he was going to sue the hospital and the doctor who had first seen him for their "incompetence." Despite my repeated advice to calm down, he spent the next two hours calling up legal colleagues and making arrangements for "a lawsuit that will teach these bastards a lesson." His blood pressure became quite elevated, despite attempts to bring it down with medication. An hour later, still talking on the telephone, the patient had his third episode of chest pains. This time, he died immediately. The autopsy revealed myocardial rupture, literally a tear in the weakened or damaged portion of his heart. This patient's rapid deterioration and eventual death were brought on directly by his thoughts.

Case No. 4

Mr. Casey, a sixty-four-year-old insurance salesman with a history of heavy smoking came to me for a routine physical examination. He had no symptoms of disease and felt perfectly well, but because of his smoking, I ordered a chest x-ray to be taken. It revealed a large lesion in the lower lobe of the left lung. Further testing disclosed that the lesion was consistent with a diagnosis of lung cancer. A later examination of an x-ray taken five years before showed a small, coin-sized lesion in the same area, suggesting that the cancer had been growing slowly for at least the previous five years. In any case, the patient had been totally free of symptoms up to the present time. After Mr. Casey heard his diagnosis, however, his condition suddenly and rapidly deteriorated. Within three days he was coughing up blood, and in three weeks he developed a severe, uncontrollable cough and shortness of breath. He died from lung cancer one month later.

This case history bears out what I have frequently observed, that a rapid progression of symptoms and then death from cancer occurred *after the diagnosis of cancer was made*. It is almost as if the patient was dying from the *diagnosis* and not from the disease. This is the placebo effect in reverse, we could say, because the causation originates in the thought, "I have cancer, therefore I am dying." The thought becomes translated via the psychophysiological connection into a sequence of pathological changes in the patient's body, and he begins to decline rapidly.

Case No. 5

Mrs. Di Angelo, sixty-three years old, was admitted to the hospital with jaundice. Jaundice is most noticeable as a yellowing of the skin and the whites of the eyes, which in this case was thought to be the result of gallstones. The patient therefore was scheduled to be taken to the operating room for surgery. When her abdomen was opened, we discovered that she did not have gallstones, but a gallbladder cancer. The cancer involved the whole abdominal cavity and had invaded the liver. The patient was considered inoperable, and without any further maneuvers we closed up the abdomen. While Mrs. Di Angelo was still in the recovery room, I informed her daughter of the diagnosis. She insisted that I not tell her mother: "I know my mother. She will die immediately if you tell her that she has cancer."

Reluctantly I told the patient that she indeed had had gallstones, which we had removed. I rationalized that her daughter would tell her the truth sometime after they went home. I also believed that the patient would not live more than a couple of months.

I next saw her eight months later in my office. Her jaundice had cleared up completely, and she looked radiant and healthy. There was no clinical evidence of any cancer. Mrs. Di Angelo still visits me regularly for routine checkups and is free of disease. The last time she came to see me, she said, "Doctor, when you admitted me to the hospital three years ago with jaundice, I was sure I had cancer. I was so relieved when you operated and found gallstones that *I made up my mind never to be sick again.*"

This is one of the most amazing cases that I have ever encountered. The placebo in this case was not a drug, but the operation. Although clinically useless, the surgery had led to a complete cure. Of course in actuality it was not even the operation, but the patient's thoughts afterward that made her live.

Case No. 6

Mr. Keller, a fifty-four-year-old businessman, was admitted to the hospital with a bleeding duodenal ulcer for the third time in three years. Careful inspection of his medical history revealed that all three episodes of bleeding had taken place in the month of April. It turned out that Mr. Keller, like everybody else, did not like paying his taxes. When I questioned him, he admitted that tax time was very stressful for him. It also turned out that he was used to making a "few justifiable adjustments" here and there in his reported income on the order of several thousand dollars, enough to save him a little in taxes. These "adjustments" were also enough, however, to cause feelings of guilt and apprehension. As in many patients prone to ulcers, Mr. Keller's unhappiness with himself was translated by his body into a physical symptom — his stomach began literally to digest itself.

When the obvious cause of his bleeding ulcer was explained to him, the patient decided that it was not worth it to continue as he had. He turned his tax affairs over to an accountant and also instructed him to make contributions to the anonymous fund that the Internal Revenue Service maintains for just such people. Since then Mr. Keller has paid a few thousand dollars more in taxes, but he saves several thousand more in reduced hospital bills, and he enjoys much better health.

This was not an extraordinary case, since the connection between leading a stressful life and developing ulcers has been known for a long time. But only recently have researchers confirmed that anxious *thoughts* by themselves can trigger excessive gastric juices, leading to ulcer attacks. Dr. Herbert Weiner, a specialist commenting on the finding that "meaningful events" can trigger ulcers, asked why such a finding was not confirmed earlier. His own answer is that since physicians do not know the exact mechanism in the body that turns meaningful events into disease symptoms, they tend to disbelieve that it happens. Another reason is that investigators look for "a common series of events or a single emotional response that perturbs all such patients." But naturally enough, ulcer patients lead quite different lives from one another and experience quite individual life events. The conclusion Dr. Weiner draws — and I entirely agree with him — is that the outside event is not the significant cause, "rather it is the meaning of the event to the person who experiences it." As scientific medicine is presently set up, much that is utterly obvious about the psychophysiological connection is overlooked because, in Dr. Weiner's words again, "no test instrument has yet been devised that admits reliable information about the meaning of an event to a person."

Yet that is precisely what ties all these case histories together.

Case No. 7

I had just started my practice in a community twenty miles north of Boston. I had joined a group of internists, two of whom subspecialized in cardiology. One Sunday evening it was my turn to be on call for all my partners. I was driving from one hospital after finishing my rounds there to another about five miles away when I received a message on my beeper to call a Mrs. Johnson immediately. She was at an extension phone located in one of the large teaching hospitals in Boston. The service operator seemed to have a certain urgency in her voice, so I stopped at the nearest pay phone to call. The voice at the other end of the line was hysterical.

"Dr. Chopra," she said, "my husband is booked for a coronary bypass operation here tomorrow, and at the last minute he wants to sign himself out!" Mrs. Johnson was talking to me because her husband was a patient of one of the cardiologists who was a senior partner of mine. Mr. Johnson suffered from unstable angina pectoris. Fearing that he might suffer a massive heart attack if surgery was not performed immediately, my partner had transferred him to the teaching hospital for an emergency heart bypass graft. The hospital to which he had been transferred was one of the most

famous in the world, and the procedure was to be performed by
Dr. W., a world-famous cardiac surgeon.

"Why does your husband want to sign himself out?" I asked
Mrs. Johnson.

"Because he doesn't like Dr. W."

"What didn't he like about Dr. W.?" I asked.

To which she replied, "Nothing in particular, he just doesn't
like him."

"Mrs. Johnson," I said impatiently, "people come from all over
the world to be operated on by Dr. W. He is famous for his skill,
and the hospital your husband is in is one of the most famous in
the world. Sheiks from the Middle East, Hollywood stars, and
heads of state fly here for treatment. Fewer than one percent of
patients who undergo the procedure your husband is scheduled to
have die from surgery. Without surgery, however, the prognosis is
dismal. Your husband is having unstable angina and is bound to
have a severe heart attack, the mortality rate from which is very
much higher than one percent. If your husband wants to sign
himself out, that is his business. But he should have a better reason than the fact that he doesn't *like* Dr. W."

Mrs. Johnson then asked anxiously if she could speak directly
with Dr. F., the partner of mine who was the cardiologist and her
husband's actual physician, not me.

"My husband knows Dr. F.," she said, "and he would listen to
him. My husband has nothing against Dr. W.; in fact, Dr. W. was
very nice to him and explained everything about the surgery very
patiently. It's just that my husband didn't like him personally —
you know, it is just a feeling."

I was running out of time; I had to get to the emergency room of
the other hospital, and I could not understand what she was trying
to tell me.

"It is Dr. F.'s night off," I said impatiently. "I think he is away
for the weekend anyway. I think your husband is lucky to be at
this hospital under such excellent care. Dr. F. went to a great deal
of trouble to arrange for his surgery, and I think your husband
should go through with it, or else he will almost certainly find

himself in big trouble. If you will excuse me now, I have to hang up. I have an emergency to attend to."

The next morning I reported this conversation to my senior partner. As I was telling him the story, he started to rush to the telephone.

"Where are you going?" I asked.

"To call off the surgery," he said. "You will learn, Deepak — never send a patient to surgery if he does not trust his surgeon." He remained on the phone for a while and then hung up. "Too late; he's already in the operating room."

That evening the famous surgeon called up my partner with bad news. An unforeseen and very rare complication had occurred as they were getting ready to take Mr. Johnson off the cardiac pump. Despite very vigorous attempts at resuscitation, he had died on the operating table.

Case No. 8

As a fourth-year medical student in India, I was once assigned to do a clinical workup on a patient with terminal cancer of the pancreas. He was a seventy-year-old villager named Laxman Govindass. Besides being quite ill, he was confused and somewhat in awe at finding himself in a large modern hospital with sophisticated machinery and teams of serious-faced physicians in long white coats. The doctors who attended him were professional academic types who spent an hour at a time by his bedside discussing with interns and residents the pathogenesis of pancreatic carcinoma and its various clinical presentations. They would then move on to the next case, sometimes without so much as asking Mr. Govindass how he felt. The interns and residents took competent care of his medical problems, but they were too busy to talk to him personally.

As a medical student assigned three workups a week, I had plenty of time to talk. In a couple of days we became very good friends. I learned that he was a farmer from a nearby district, that he had three grown sons who now looked after the farm, that he had previously been a very heavy drinker, and because of the drinking his family had forsaken and finally deserted him. When he became critically ill, one of his sons brought him to this hospital and said farewell with the words, "You will probably die!"

Naturally, the patient felt bewildered at being in the hospital, and now without the numbing effects of alcohol, he suddenly became aware of the searing pain in his abdomen. For the first time he realized how sick he really was. His condition deteriorated rapidly, and his pain grew worse. He found the doctors more interested in his disease than in him. With no family to comfort him, he soon began to wish that he would just die.

I spent an hour or so with him every evening, often without much exchange in the way of words. It was abundantly clear to both of us that he had very little time left. Then my clinical routine came to an end. I was assigned to a village posting, a small infirmary about two hundred miles away. I went to wish Mr. Govindass goodbye, knowing full well that he would not be alive in a month when I returned to the hospital.

I kept a stiff upper lip, however, and said, "Mr. Govindass, I will see you when I return in thirty days."

He smiled sadly and said, "Now that you are leaving, I have nothing to live for; I will die." He was already moribund and emaciated and weighed no more than seventy-five pounds. It was a wonder he was alive.

Not knowing what else to say, I muttered, "Don't be silly. You cannot die before I see you again."

I left for my village posting. The dispensary to which I was assigned turned out to be grossly understaffed, and I was kept busy doing what really needed four men. I am ashamed to say that I seldom thought of my dying friend back in the hospital. When I returned a month later, I had almost forgotten about him. Outside the ward, though, I saw the name Laxman Govindass, and my heart started beating violently. I broke out in a cold sweat; I could not believe that he was still alive. I rushed to his bedside. The old man lay crouched in bed in a fetal pose. He was nothing but skin and bone, except for one striking aspect — the large, bulging eyes that pierced me and looked deep into the innermost recesses of my soul.

"You have come back," he said. "You said I could not die without seeing you again. I am seeing you now!" He closed his eyes and with one breath was gone.

I was deeply shaken. I could not forgive myself for prolonging this man's final agony. I felt wretched and guilty, and many a night I woke up to find myself staring into his accusing eyes.

I will never forget Laxman Govindass. It was through him that I stumbled upon the psychophysiological connection.

II

Laying the Foundation

Let noble thoughts come to us from every side.

— Rig Veda

14

All Health Originates in One Place

BY NOW the reader should be well aware of the hypothesis I am developing. The evidence for it is unmistakable. We have dealt with common but serious problems such as high blood pressure, heart disease, cancer, overweight, chronic fatigue, depression, burned-out syndrome, and psychiatric illness. We have found that the mind has a crucial role to play in the genesis of all these disorders. In my view, this will be true of any other disease one looks at as well. Ulcers occur in uptight, anxious people. Ulcerative colitis, a painful intestinal disorder, afflicts people who are compulsive and obsessive. Impotence and various other sexual problems are almost always due to performance anxiety. Accidents happen most often to people who are habitually prone to them, who have a characteristic absent-mindedness that attracts mishaps.

We could go on to discuss numerous other well-documented examples. As we probe deeper into the pathogenesis of disease, however, a primary truth comes to light: all disease results from the disruption of the flow of intelligence. When people speak of intelligence, they refer almost automatically to the intellect and its dealing in concepts. Intelligence is not simply in the head, though.

Its expression may be at the subcellular level, at the cellular or tissue level, or at the level of the central nervous system. Enzymes, genes, receptors, antibodies, hormones, and neurons are expressions of intelligence.

And they *possess* an intelligence. They regulate essential functions with perfect know-how and do it at the body's far outposts, so to speak, far from the castle where intellect is seated. Although all these expressions of intelligence can be located, intelligence itself cannot. It permeates each level of its expression; it is all-pervasive in us and universal in nature. Intelligence is mind, and, as we shall see, its scope embraces the cosmos. We would be rash to suppose that it operates from the confines of the brain alone. In that sense, all disease processes originate on this vaster stage of Mind.

So also does health.

15

Happiness and the Brain Chemistry of Health

IT IS QUITE OBVIOUS that healthy people are happier than unhealthy people. What is now becoming increasingly evident
through study is that the reverse is also true: happy people are
healthier than unhappy people. It appears that happiness, which
simply means having happy thoughts most of the time, causes biochemical changes in the brain that in turn have profoundly beneficial effects on the body's physiology.

Sad or depressing thoughts, on the other hand, produce changes
in brain chemistry that have a detrimental effect on the body's
physiology. The brain chemicals through which thoughts are
working are called neuro-transmitters. At least thirty different
kinds of them have been identified in brain tissue. According to
the mood that a person has cultivated, the ratio of these neuro-
transmitters to one another changes. Since thoughts are under
our conscious control — we can consciously choose to think any
particular thought — it becomes obvious that brain chemistry,
though it may be difficult to analyze scientifically, can be controlled very easily. To think is to practice brain chemistry.
The chemistry influences hormone secretion from various sites

throughout the brain, such as the hypothalamus and the pituitary, and these hormones then carry messages to distant organs in the body.

Let us take a few specific examples, first, of unhappy thoughts. Angry, hostile thoughts bring about rapid heartbeat, a rise in blood pressure, and flushing of the face, among other changes. Anxious thoughts can also speed up the heart and raise blood pressure, as well as induce tremor of the hands, cold sweat, a knotted stomach, and a pervasive weakening, as when we say a person is "sick with dread." Different kinds of thoughts must produce chemical changes in the brain in order to account for such physical manifestations. Severely disturbed thought has long been linked to distortions in brain chemistry. To quote one researcher, "There is no twisted thought without a twisted molecule."

Likewise, happy thoughts of all kinds, loving thoughts, thoughts of peace and tranquillity, of compassion, friendliness, kindness, generosity, affection, warmth, and intimacy each produce a corresponding state of physiology via the flux of neuro-transmitters and hormones in the central nervous system. The profound physiological changes that happy thoughts induce lead to good health because the neuro-transmitters that mediate them in the body have a stimulating effect. If, as we have seen, the body's immune system is weakened by feelings of anger, apathy, enmity, resentment, conflict, and gloom, then happy thought patterns should serve to increase the body's resistance to disease through a similar, but reversed effect.

One sees just this in the "placebo effect," whereby thoughts alone determine the outcome of a disease process. A placebo is a pill made of nothing but sugar and some inert coloring to make it look like an authentic drug. Patients are given it with the information that it is in fact an authentic and powerful medicine, usually a painkiller. Entirely because the patients expect relief — the word *placebo* is Latin for "I shall please" — relief comes. For example, in one recent study members of a group of patients suffering from bleeding ulcers were given what their doctors described as the most potent current drug for treating ulcers. The ulcers of more than 70 percent immediately stopped bleeding. Another group, however, was told that the drug was experimental and therefore unknown in its efficacy; the ulcers of only 25 percent stopped bleeding in this group. In reality neither group took anything but a placebo.

The ramifications of such researches go far beyond what was previously imagined. In the past it was thought that the placebo effect took the place of "real" treatment by more or less fooling the patient, or rather by having him fool himself. Doctors recognized that placebos worked, but their action seemed a curious psychological side effect. Now we know that placebos induce the body's own healing mechanisms (I have already described a whole class of internal painkillers, the endorphins, which the body manufactures for this purpose). If we look ahead far enough, we can see that placebos may be the best medicine of all. I look upon them as a kind of permission that the mind gives to itself so that healing can take place. Researchers are beginning to see the possibilities of employing the placebo effect in the treatment of serious organic diseases, including cancer. Norman Cousins, whose books have awakened the public to such possibilities, writes, "The placebo, then, is not so much a pill as a process. . . . The placebo is the doctor who resides within."

Placebos work through the release of neuro-transmitters. This means in effect that it is not the placebo but the thought of the patient taking the placebo that is the active agent. In the ulcer study, the patients stopped bleeding because of their *belief* that the drug would work, and the weaker the belief, the weaker the cure. Placebos are so powerful when they do work that in one study patients were relieved of nausea when given a pill they were told was a powerful antinausea drug. In fact the pill was a powerful drug to *induce* nausea. When belief is channeled in one direction, the "reality" of a drug's action can be completely changed, not simply enhanced. A belief that a pill will cure headaches, relieve pain, lower blood pressure, improve sexual ability, increase strength and vitality, improve appetite, put on or take off weight, or even cure a malignancy can bring about that very result.

For thoughts to be capable of curing, they must be innocently held and sincerely believed in over a period of time, because the longer the curative thought patterns influence the appropriate neuro-transmitters, the more the neuro-transmitters can influence the physiology of the brain. If thought patterns and our state of mind are so important, how can we change them for the better? To answer this question, we first have to understand what a thought is and what we mean by *mind*. That is the subject of the next chapter.

16

Thoughts, Impulses of Intelligence —
The Human Mind, a Reservoir
of Intelligence

THIS BOOK you are reading now is nothing but an outpouring of thoughts from my mind streaming through your senses into your mind. Look around and you will see thoughts in manifestation everywhere. The chair you are sitting in had its origin in a thought, like the house or apartment you live in, the bed you sleep in, the clothes you wear, the car you drive, the food you eat, the work you do. There really can be no argument about this obvious fact: whatever you can perceive around you that human beings have made — highways, cars, jets, spaceships, computers, Gothic novels, jellybeans — is nothing but manifested thoughts, some your own, the vast majority from people you do not know, but thoughts nevertheless. Maharishi Mahesh Yogi, an authority on consciousness and a great explainer of it, calls thoughts "impulses of creative intelligence." These impulses arise naturally and in unlimited supply from the mind, which is therefore the reservoir of creative intelligence. When thoughts, or impulses of creative intelligence, are organized well enough, they easily lead to creative action, and from action we have the outward manifestations of books, objects, and healthy bodies.

The route that leads from consciousness to created things is in our experience all the time; we just do not consciously pay attention to it. Once we do pay attention to it, however, a wider view of life opens up. For example, let us say I am an artist. Impulses of intelligence streaming out of my consciousness — my mind — when properly organized lead to an action. I gather raw materials, paintbrushes, paint, and begin to mix them in an organized way. The result will be a new thing created by my thought, a painting. In order for the painting to appear on the scene, a few things are utterly indispensable: (a) consciousness, or mind, from which will arise (b) thoughts, or impulses of creative intelligence; they come out (c) in an organized manner that leads to (d) an action, and the crowning glory is (e) my painting — a moderately satisfying picture of the Taj Mahal by moonlight.

The ability to organize thoughts is just as innate as the thoughts themselves or the fact that they are intelligent. Any activity of life that is not random — and no creative act is random in all of nature — carries with it, just when it is born, the power to organize. When an architect draws up a blueprint, each line of his carries with it the ability actually to be built. This innate organizing power Maharishi calls "knowledge." Ideas could not turn into things as naturally as they do if they did not contain knowledge. We overlook organizing power because it is so well embedded in our intelligence. When the mind wants the hand to make a fist, the response from the hand is automatic, but it takes an entire course on physiology to explain the knowledge that runs silently from brain to hand via the know-how of neuro-transmitters, hormones, electrical charges, enzymes, and muscle actions, not to mention the ongoing intelligence that maintains the life and nourishment of brain and hands. In fact, we can define mind as that structure that has organizing power.

What about objects that are not manmade, the objects of nature? These fall for us into two categories, living and nonliving. Not that every culture sees plants and animals as alive and fire, earth, and wind as not alive, but we can consider them that way. Among living things, science now admits that no level is without intelligence. The span of organizing power arches from the brain to the nucleus of every cell. At the moment of our conception, the single-celled fertilized ovum is nothing except a set of instructions coded on a molecule of double-stranded DNA. The instructions are bound up in an organized manner, the unfolding expression of which leads to a specific human being. If the DNA unfolds as Albert Einstein, then this ability to change the world through thoughts will move an infinite distance. It will move from organized biochemicals in one cell to the infinitely creative mind of Einstein. We are seeing that life has infinite organizing power, or knowledge, built into it.

Let us take the nonliving objects of nature. Take a piece of rock and break it down — crack it, powder it, purify its basic chemicals, then smash the chemicals into atoms and shatter the atoms into elementary particles — then what do we see? We see organization. We see protons, electrons, and other particles arranged in an organized manner. Before the cracking, blasting, powdering, and smashing, this knowledge went about its existence coherently, automatically, and, we can say, intelligently. All nonliving objects express their own variety of know-how in the scheme of nature.

The point I am trying to make is this: Everything we comprehend in the universe with our senses — that is, all objects man-made or natural, living or nonliving — are expressions of organizing power, or knowledge. Another insight from Maharishi Mahesh Yogi comes to mind: "Knowledge is structured in consciousness." We have already seen how this idea applies to our minds. Every impulse flowing from a human mind — consciousness — carries knowledge with it. But the concept actually launches out into the universe. Einstein himself remarked that all science begins in "a deep conviction of the rationality of the universe." He described his feelings of "rapturous amazement at the harmony of natural law," and one of his primary convictions was that such harmony pointed to an intelligence of the utmost superiority which the universe displays. One of the most famous pieces of Indian wisdom from the Vedas is the sentence, "I am That, Thou art That, all this is That, and That alone is." We will not think of this as a mystic riddle once we see that the word "That" means "intelligence."

All things in the universe, then, arise from consciousness as knowledge. This is an astonishing concept to grasp and come to terms with. It tells us that the only thing in the universe that is real and tangible is knowledge. This knowledge (or organizing power) has its seat in consciousness, and all the rest of the material world is by comparison not as real. Material things have their own undeniable reality in the order of things — the stars, rocks, mushrooms, and kangaroos are out there — but when we trace them back upstream to their source, they are manifestations of the one primary reality, which is knowledge. Napoleon Hill, who has developed an approach to success in life based on this concept, writes, "We look not to the things that are seen, but to the things that are unseen, for the things that are seen are transient, but the things that are unseen are eternal."

Let me restate what has been said on a practical level. First, we have consciousness, in which reside all the impulses of creative intelligence. These are expressed as thoughts in our minds. When expressed in an organized manner — via organizing power, or knowledge — they lead to action and result in material creation. This process taking place in us is paralleled throughout nature on a universal scale. Our impulses are the same as all the other impulses of intelligence. We just call them thoughts because that is how we think of them. A bird in mid-Atlantic flight also has an impulse of intelligence to guide it, leading to the action of its migration (including all the prior actions of stocking up on food, choosing the right season for migrating, and so on). That impulse in the bird's brain is also a thought of a sort, only we do not call it one because we are accustomed to thinking of thoughts only in human terms. We could just as easily say that *thoughts* guide a bee to gather pollen and make honey if we were accustomed to say so.

All of nature, therefore, is nothing but a teeming universe of all kinds of impulses or thoughts expressing themselves in the infinite variety of creation.

So also when we look to our bodies. We see the same infinite intelligence in operation. Only, we are used to thinking of intelligence as residing just in the brain; this is because we are used to equating intelligence with intellectual capacity. However, with our new insight we discover intelligence operating in every cell of our body. The intricate machinery of the heart, the kidney, the immune or hormone system — all these are other expressions of organizing power. We come to the inescapable conclusion that mind or consciousness or intelligence pervades every part of the created universe. Our own minds are an expression of this intelligence; from it our human consciousness derives its infinite scope.

17

Evolution

SOME YEARS AGO, an infinite amount of information packaged in a minuscule, flagellating, single-celled sperm was combined with an infinite amount of information packaged in a single-celled microscopic ovum. The result was again an infinite amount of information, now packaged in an infinitesimally small, single-celled conceptus. That conceptus was unique, because there was nothing exactly like it in the entire universe — it alone possessed that package of infinite information coded into a double strand of DNA. With proper conditions and food, the cell divided again and again, billions of times, all the time carrying with it its unique knowledge and its unique packet of information. Today that cell is billions of cells, working in concert with each other in a display of knowledge and intelligence that never loses its intricate powers of organization. Today that cell is you.

It is not just your substance. It is all of your thoughts, your emotions, likes, dislikes, desires, and passions. Today you may be captaining an enterprise or looking up at the evening star from a rowboat, reading Greek or stirring up a revolution. You may turn out a Hitler or a Gandhi, and the world may think different thoughts because you lived in it. Who are you? In truth you are none other than that single cell, accidentally engendered when one of several hundred million sperm cells, carrying its unique set of instructions, surging ahead of its companions, entered an ovum in your mother's womb.

The code of instructions on that double strand of DNA is the same today as it was then. In a real sense you are just that set of instructions and nothing else. It is all of you — your skin, your eyes, your senses, your mind, your intellect. You are *a piece of knowledge*. That knowledge continues to be expressed in infinite variety, so you are not the same person today as you were yesterday, and you will be an utterly different person tomorrow. The flow of change is made possible by what appears to be its opposite, the changeless code packaged in your DNA. When the two opposites work together, change and nonchange produce continuous growth. That is what we call evolution.

Evolution does not mean that you have become different or acquired more knowledge. The knowledge was complete and whole to begin with. It was infinite when it started out as the stored information of a single cell. It is only that the expression of that knowledge is ever expanding. Is there a limit to this expansion and therefore to evolution? The focus of science on the material world may lead us to think that evolution is basically a stepladder for primitive organisms to climb until they "finish" their development as the species of plants and animals on earth. Science is on the verge of understanding evolution as much more than that, however.

Evolution is the nature of life. Let me quote the eminent physician and researcher Jonas Salk:

> The principle of evolution that must be kept in mind is that it permeates everything. Before biological evolution, there was an antecedent pre-biological evolution; before that there was the evolution of the cosmos. After biological evolution there was metabiological evolution, the evolution of consciousness, and of consciousness of consciousness, as well as consciousness of evolution. Evolution is taking place within the human mind right now as a result of human experi-

ence, which we metabolize, which becomes incorporated into our being. Human thought and human creativity have all developed in response to human environment. Metabiological evolution involves survival of the wisest. Wisdom is now becoming the new criterion of fitness.

Dr. Salk is telling us that the goal of evolution in man is "survival of the wisest." We have been brought to this point by evolution itself, the same tendency that formed the stars, the earth, and life on earth. At all of these stages, the operation of evolution is effortless. It is simply in the nature of existence to grow. Growing wise will simply be the next stage of growth. We do not have to *do* anything except follow the natural tendency that made us conscious in the first place, then conscious of being conscious in the second place.

If wisdom is the criterion for survival, then what is wisdom? In India the classic definition of a wise man is "a knower of reality." We could say that wisdom is knowing about life as a whole. As human intelligence effortlessly expands, we come to understand life as a whole — that is why we are so interested in perfect health and happiness. These are the natural, evolving goals of people who begin to grasp the infinite intelligence expressed in their minds and bodies. Once we accept that our natural tendency is to expand in knowledge, then the next step is to show why the goal of this expansion is increased happiness.

18

Health — The Sum of Positive and Negative Impulses of Intelligence

AT ANY ONE TIME, your health is the sum total of all the impulses, positive and negative, emanating from your consciousness. You are what you think. If you are happy, this just means that you have happy thoughts most of the time. If you are depressed, it means that you have sad thoughts most of the time. Into this calculation enter all our other states of mind as well, our daily share of anger, fear, envy, greed, kindness, compassion, benevolence, and love. These are all simply thoughts. When one of them happens to predominate, it leads to a corresponding state of mind and, as we have seen, to a corresponding state of physiology.

In fact, we can restate the evidence for the psychophysiological connection in one sentence: For every state of consciousness, there is a corresponding state of physiology. If you are having hostile thoughts, for example, they will be reflected in your mood, your facial expression, your social behavior, and how you feel physically. You scowl, you are impatient and difficult to deal with, you churn up too much acid in your stomach and a lot of adrenaline in your blood stream, and consequently you may develop peptic ulcers and hypertension. For an observant person, it is not at all difficult literally to read your thoughts. And the cells of your body are registering them far more accurately.

In most people, the psychophysiological connection operates more or less randomly. Thoughts arise from interactions with the world, these thoughts affect the body for better or worse, and they leave a lingering impression in the form of moods, tendencies toward disease, actual disease symptoms, and the process of wearing out the body over time, which we call aging. Very little of this is under our conscious control. However, it is obvious that *some* thoughts are under our control, and this simple fact leaves an opening for further growth in the proper direction, toward mastery of the self.

Mastery of the self has classically been called "enlightenment." Since this concept is quite badly understood in our society, we will discuss it in detail later on. But enlightenment simply means having control over the psychophysiological connection. The highly evolved mind is not a prey to random influences of ill health; it has mastery over what it thinks. Therefore, what it thinks is happy and healthy. Mastery of this kind is not something peculiar or "not normal." It is simply an *extension* of the normal ability to control *some* thoughts. This natural capacity, when given room to expand and evolve, goes in one direction, and that is toward more perfect health and greater happiness. That is what Dr. Salk meant by survival of the wisest.

Because it is in the nature of life to evolve, we do not have to *do* anything to evolve in the proper direction. Gaining mastery of the self, with all its benefits to health, means little more than stepping out of the way and allowing the infinite intelligence of the mind and body to cooperate more fully. That is what they want to do. When we stop interfering and are wise enough to let the psychophysiological connection work for us instead of against us, our minds rush as quickly as possible toward perfect health.

19

Living and Longevity —
The Problem of Aging

AGING IS the progressive deterioration of physical and mental functioning that occurs with time, ending with the cessation of all function, which is death. The mechanics of aging are not clear. Until recently, scientists had not shown much interest in the aging process, and not too much long-term research on it exists. However, the function of the separate organs in the body has been clearly studied, and there is only one way to describe how they age: they progressively decline over time. Hormones also have been studied, and researchers have found that interesting changes occur in the concentration of them in the blood, particularly the pituitary and adrenal hormones. As people grow older, there is a rise in their blood of a pituitary hormone called thyroid-stimulating hormone (TSH) and a fall in the concentration of an adrenal hormone called dehydroepiandrosterone sulfate. (Not that you should remember this name. I know it because I was involved in some of this research.) The reversal of these levels, which has important implications for the reversal of aging, is discussed in part IV of this book.

Some recent animal research, which may or may not apply

equally well to humans, casts further light on the mechanics of aging. It was found, for example, that periodic fasting increases the life span of rats. Fasting has traditionally been a part of many cultures and figures in most religions; our morning meal, for example, is called "breakfast" because there was once a fast to break. If fasting does prove to have a physiological benefit, this proof could be connected to the observation that fasting raises the level of growth hormone secreted by the pituitary.

One effect of growth hormone is to stimulate the production of T-lymphocytes from the thymus gland; these play an important role in keeping up the body's immunity to disease. Aging and age-related diseases like arthritis occur when the body's immune response is weakened. It is also now known that physical exercise raises the level of growth hormone too. Objective science thus supports the claim of many lay people that regular exercise and fasting are measures that prolong life. Getting a good night's sleep has long been thought to help one live longer, and it turns out that the level of growth hormone rises during sleep as well. The amino acids arginine and ornithine have the same effect; that is why health food stores around the country are selling them now as "youth pills," backed by the popular writing on life extension.

It is too early to tell whether the attempts to increase levels of growth hormone through exercise, fasting, or supplements will really prolong one's life span, but the initial data appear promising. I should caution that fasting has drawbacks if it is carried too far, including protein-calorie malnourishment and weakening of the immune system. By and large, the dietary measures agreed on by most authorities in the field follow these guidelines: Reduce the amount you eat gradually over a period of several weeks, avoid all processed foods, avoid foods high in fat, salt, and sugar, and concentrate on increasing the amount of fresh fruits and vegetables in the diet. Once you have adjusted to these changes, you can begin fasts by skipping one meal in the day or by just drinking milk or juice in place of a meal. If you fast for an entire day, then once a week is enough.

"Life extension" advice has also touched on substances in the diet called antioxidants. It is thought that aging and age-related disease processes like hardening of the arteries may occur because "free radicals" are formed in the body. Free radicals are highly reactive substances that create abnormal chemical bonds in body tissue; they result from interactions between our cells and outside agents taken in through polluted air, cigarette smoke, impure water, and certain foods. Oxygen is used up during these reactions. We are advised to take in antioxidants because they prevent the formation of these free radicals by prohibiting the oxygen from binding chemically.

Many of these antioxidants are found in natural foods, but the "life extension" plan tells you to boost them with supplements. The ones generally available in health food stores include vitamins A, C, and E, pantothenic acid, and the food preservatives BHT and BHA. It is also easy to buy the trace minerals zinc and selenium, and the amino acids cysteine, ornithine, and arginine, which are recommended as well. Since this is quite a cloudy area, I am not passing on the dosages advised by the "life extension" program nor am I endorsing these recommendations. Food preservatives have known toxic effects, for one thing, and the shift from wanting food with "no preservatives" marked on the label to wanting to buy preservative capsules simply shows that our knowledge here is inconclusive. Proponents of vitamin E have claimed for a long time that it has beneficial effects in retarding aging, but even if that is agreed upon — and not all researchers are convinced — the optimal dosage is far from settled.

Emotional stress and worry can hasten the aging process. Working through the neuro-endocrine axis that we are now familiar with in this book, stressful thoughts are translated into neurotransmitters in the brain. These in turn affect the concentration of "stress hormones" such as ACTH in the pituitary. When the whole hormonal sequence is triggered, the result is a weakening of the immune system, or immunosuppression, and, as we have discussed already, when the immune response is suppressed, the body becomes much more susceptible to disease of all kinds, including cancer. Therefore, it is felt that the benefits of stress reduction include the enhancing of our chances to live longer.

Longevity and Intelligence

As interesting as the biochemistry of aging is proving to be, I think it is more fruitful to look deeper. To begin with, once they realized that the central nervous system plays a critical part in aging, researchers began to hypothesize that aging is a preset mechanism. This theory arises because it is well known that our DNA programs many of our life events "on time," including when we teethe and when we enter puberty. Also, it was discovered that the amount of natural antioxidants produced by the body is largely determined by heredity; this helps us to understand why certain gene pools of people may enjoy great longevity, with members consistently living past eighty years of age.

The theory, then, is that the brain has a built-in biological clock that determines life span. The maximum life span for the species would be determined by this clock, and environmental factors will affect it only if they are of specific kinds. The clock operates in animals besides man; for instance, the life cycle of the salmon ends soon after it has swum upstream to spawn, a preset function in the central nervous system of each fish. The setting of the biological clock is determined genetically, and this finding has opened exciting possibilities for genetic manipulation, often called genetic engineering, that would have the specific effect of prolonging life. Essentially this involves changing the coding in the DNA so that the clock would be reset. The possibility of creating immortal cells from the genetic level is stimulating the imagination of biologists in the field. Already the techniques exist to "immortalize" cells in a test tube — in other words, these cells will live forever.

Immortality is not new to nature, however. The lowly amoeba, one of the most familiar of one-celled organisms, is physically immortal in a quite literal sense. When one amoeba grows too old, it divides into two younger, more vibrant amoebae. The original amoeba does not die; it turns into its two daughters. And as they mature, they will do the same. In this continual, everlasting propagation of new generations, the first amoeba still remains — no corpse is ever found. Another primitive organism found in water, the hydra, has reached everlasting life by another means. Its metabolism is so rapid that all of its body cells are replaced every two weeks. Its life expectancy thus remains a constant; there is no aging for a hydra and no death.

Nature's intelligence has programmed other cold-blooded species — certain types of fish and crocodiles — with such low metabolic rates that their cells are forever growing. These creatures keep on maturing forever with no fixed adult size, and death befalls them only when they become prey for other predators. Among plants, the sequoias and bristlecone pines may not be immortal, but some are alive and well at ages of between two thousand and five thousand years. The bodhi tree under which the Buddha meditated three thousand years ago still stands as a shrine and place of pilgrimage in India today.

When scientists attempt to "immortalize" cells using the techniques of microengineering, they are not altering the actual content of the genes but merely the expression of that content. Genes themselves have always known the secret of immortality. They are the one living entity within us that never dies. Mutations may occur to change the expression of genes over the millennia, but the genes themselves live on forever.

This fact was brought home to me rather dramatically fourteen years ago when my wife was pregnant with our first child. A routine blood test revealed that she was mildly anemic. I assumed that she had a mild iron deficiency, but out of curiosity I examined through a microscope the slide prepared from a drop of Rita's blood. When I saw some peculiar shapes in her red blood cells, I consulted the pathologist at our hospital, who immediately pronounced a diagnosis of "mild Mediterranean anemia." A more sophisticated blood test revealed that Rita had the thalassemia minor trait, as he had said.

Thalassemia is a blood disorder common to Mediterranean

peoples, but my wife comes from New Delhi and has no known relatives outside that part of India. I went to the library and made inquiries of epidemiologists and researchers in India and so discovered that a "belt of thalassemia" ran all the way from Macedonia in the north of Greece to a region called Multan in what is now Pakistan. It turns out that Rita's great-grandfather immigrated to India from Multan. Moreover, the "belt of thalassemia" roughly traces the campaigns of Alexander the Great along the route his armies took more than three centuries before the birth of Christ.

As I sat there for the hundredth time looking at this little smear of blood through my microscope, seated in the dingy laboratory of a community hospital in New Jersey, the reality of immortality dawned on me with a sudden feeling of exhilaration. The genes coursing through my wife's veins in all their casualness had outlived all — Alexander dejected on the banks of the Indus, the Sermon on the Mount, the destruction of Pompeii, the Crusades, Napoleon's retreat from Moscow, centuries of revolution, and the tide of affairs that no man and only a few ideas have outlasted — those genes I was staring at had persisted unchanged while all else had succumbed to change. They had survived the upheavals of the centuries, they continued to survive in my wife, and now they have passed on to my children. Surely we need no more convincing proof of immortality — genes are its living embodiment.

Should we think of genes as physical structures or as unique expressions of knowledge, impulses of intelligence? They are both. They are physical, because you can see them and analyze their structure in terms of chemical components, but like other living tissue, genes transcend their merely physical nature. Their existence is always in a dynamic relationship with nature as a whole. They are caught up in the same flow of evolution that upholds the universe, whether on the scale of a micron or a galaxy. Genes are precipitated information. They are the physical expression in the utmost concentrated form of knowledge that has always existed. Yet they also uphold life here and now — they are nature's ultimate device for allowing the changeless to change with every moment. Like our thoughts, our genes will never be the same after the present instant, but their chemical stability allows all the myriads of instants to link together into a span of living time — a human lifetime.

Genes have found a home in our cells, but they were schooled in the cosmos. It has taken eons for the universe to "learn" how to fashion hydrogen, carbon, and other elements of the periodic chart, then to make organic molecules of increasing complexity, and finally to erect a viable setting, this planet, so that life could issue forth in unlimited freedom. All that was usefully learned, any piece of information relevant to the current end product, which is humanity, has been stored in human genes. And there is every sign that the process will continue.

So our genes have learned something of immortality. If we are to grasp immortality at other levels of our intelligence, we will have to find a mode of experience that is not bound up in either "thinking about it" or trying to see or touch it. Our everyday dependence on thinking and using the senses is permanently tied up with this thing we call time. Since aging occurs with the passing of time, we must have a clearer conception of time if we want a clearer conception of aging. J. Krishnamurti, a wise Indian thinker and teacher, has called time "the psychological enemy of man." Since we almost universally fear growing old, this seems undeniable. But what is time? Krishnamurti says simply, "Thought is time." For the patient who is experiencing the aging of his body and mind, or for the physician who treats the symptoms that are time's practical outcome in the physiology, this is a fascinating idea. It asks us to realize that time is a concept.

In *Space, Time and Medicine,* a book I highly recommend, Dr. Larry Dossey observes that

> we cling to the idea of a real time — a time that flows and is divisible into past, present, and future. Our belief in a linear real time underlies our basic assumptions of health and disease, of living and dying. But this kind of thinking is tied to an older science.

The older science he refers to was overthrown by Einstein's general theory of relativity, which forced us to regard time, space, and human sense organs as bound up in one unbroken continuum. In order to consider the "reality" of time, you must consider the consciousness that is perceiving it and the whole of nature in which both are at home. We have created time, you and I. It is a mental device, a concept we use to measure the relative positions of existing things. We must no longer think of time as an entity unto itself. It is only a partner in the space-time continuum, and specific changes in that continuum can change time. It was Einstein who first postulated that if you travel fast enough to approach the speed of light (roughly 186,000 miles per second), then you would slow down or "dilate" time. That means that if you sustained such a speed long enough to reach the nearest star and return in three years, you would find that time on the earth had measured out twenty-one years. This would be a reality for the cells of your body, which would be younger than the cells of the people who did not make the trip with you. You would have experienced aging as a relative phenomenon.

There is more here than just the riddles of high-speed physics. Dr. Dossey goes on to say that

> mortality, birth, death, longevity, illness, and health — we unconsciously construct these ideas, incorporating into them an *absolute* time which we assume to be part of an *external* reality. But if Einstein was correct that all knowledge about reality begins and ends in experience, there is no external reality from which these events draw meaning. Our knowledge of health begins and ends with experience.

Then health, illness, life, and death are not absolutes; they are bound up in us and come from us. Our way of looking at ourselves makes us what we are. If we could only change our way of looking, we could in fact change all notions and therefore all realities of living, aging, mortality, and ultimately immortality — *for it is our notions that construct those realities.* This conclusion dawns upon us once we grasp the idea that our thoughts and our way of seeing indeed structure the entire material universe.

Think of it for a moment. What is your body composed of? It is composed of tissues and cells that on a finer scale are nothing but the organized arrangement of molecules and atoms. Smaller than these are the subatomic particles that have existed since time was time. They were not created for your birth, nor will they die when your cells decompose. They form a part of the matter of the universe and therefore a part of the space-time continuum. It is only their specific arrangement now that makes up the entity that is you. In fact, the body that is yours is not even composed of the same particles today that composed it a few years ago. Thanks to the constant replacement of old cells by new ones, old matter with new matter, your body's arrangement is forever rearranging.

You should not think of your body as a "frozen sculpture," then, but as a river. Heraclitus, an ancient Greek philosopher, left us with a sentence that has described our nature for centuries: "You cannot step twice into the same river, for new water is always flowing in." The analogy with a river is particularly beautiful and apt. So long as the flow of change within us is fresh, we will be perfectly healthy. Aging is the stagnation of that flow. There is only so much you can do about the body in physical terms before you reach the point where it is necessary simply to be natural with it, which is to be wise. I think of the human physiology when I read what Hermann Hesse writes in *Siddhartha:* "Love this river, stay by it, learn from it."

Because he wanted to learn about himself, Siddhartha stayed by the river; he

wanted to learn from it, he wanted to listen to it. It seemed to him that whoever understood this river and its secrets would understand much more, many secrets, all secrets.

. . . today he saw only one of the river's secrets, one that gripped his soul. He saw that the water continually flowed and flowed and yet it was always there; it was always the same and yet every moment it was new. Who could understand, conceive this? He did not understand it; he was only aware of a dim suspicion, a faint memory, divine voices.

Like that river, your body is ever the same and yet at every moment new. You are not absolute, static matter. The matter itself was once interstellar dust, and nature has future uses for it in the cosmos. Right now, the carbon in your bones and the oxygen in your blood plasma are moving in dynamic exchange with the world through the processes of digestion, respiration, and elimination. For every atom that is at home, another is traveling, and another is waiting at the station. So if your material body does not seem to rank as the "real" you, being too much like the flux that carries water downhill and leftovers from the table to the trash heap, what is the real you?

The real you is the *arrangement,* the *organizing power,* the *knowledge,* the *intelligence,* the *impulse of consciousness* that designs material stuff to give the appearance of you. That is the only reality worthy to rank as you in your completeness. It is nonmaterial, whole, dynamic and yet utterly stable, and infinite in its capacity to evolve. Through its own infinite expression it gives the appearance of changing, evolving, declining, decaying, and dying. But essentially it stands back from the appearance of change, because intelligence controls change.

Later on we will discuss how contemporary science, through a branch called quantum physics, accounts for all this in measurable terms. For now, we only need to see that human intuition has grasped such realizations for many centuries. Speaking of man's essential nature, the ancient Bhagavad Gita declares,

> He is never born, nor does he ever die, nor having once been, does he cease to be. Unborn, eternal, everlasting, ancient, he is not slain when the body is slain. Weapons cannot cleave him, nor fire burn him; water cannot wet him, nor wind dry him away. He is eternal, all-pervading, stable, immovable, ever the same. He is declared to be unmanifest, unthinkable, unchangeable.

The *he* in this passage is intelligence. It acts as the formative force in you and therefore *is* the real you. To describe the forces that it holds to be basic in the universe, science uses the term *field.* Just as a magnetic field can organize iron filings on a sheet of paper into a specific pattern, so the universe's collective field can organize body and mind — and has. From this field spring all the impulses that are responsible for creation. Whatever lives and dies participates in this field and never leaves it. Maharishi Mahesh Yogi says of it simply that it is the "field of all possibilities."

I have taken the problem of aging this far knowing that we would wind up far beyond hormone levels and "life extension" pills. We realized early on, when we examined disease processes, that health resides at the level of the "self." Now we have arrived at the self — it is our conscious intelligence. If we employ it in the service of old assumptions built up from ages of saddened experience, then disease and aging are our inevitable lot. We would do well to inform our children of their poor inheritance if we intend to be fair to them. But I think that our current stage of evolution, what Dr. Salk introduced as survival of the wisest, will guide us to an expansion of the self instead.

This expansion will be effortless because it comes from within. But the attitude that prepares the soil for its new seed is one of willingness to grow. Disease and aging persist because of myths and prejudices that propel people into decline. Our current belief system — in other words, what we expect our bodies to do — grew through centuries of cultural conditioning and indoctrination. (Most of us, for example, can recall the shock we felt when acupuncture turned out to *work*. Weren't we certain up to then that surgery absolutely required forcible chemical anesthesia?) Our belief system has sunk its roots deep into our physiology, and so we call it "true." The common man decays and declines swiftly over time because of this "truth," while the man who manages to live long and vitally until the end is considered uncommon.

All of this can and will change because of the psychophysiological connection. Whatever our thoughts and beliefs, they are mediated through the central nervous system — that is how the old thoughts sank their roots into our cells to begin with. When the messages coming from the central nervous system are changed, then the body has no choice but to change, too. First we will have to throw out the relics and residues of outworn ideas — we must be willing to be perfectly healthy forever. With that, the combined intelligence of mind and body, relieved at their liberation, will progress to a new stage of evolution. They are tending that way now or books like this would not come to be written. The next thing to consider, then, is what our new expectations for ourselves might look like.

20

From Man to Superman

MAN HAS EVOLVED over eons of time from a single-celled organism to a creature of infinite potential. Today he stands on the threshold of ever newer and bolder discoveries. But no discovery in nature takes place without a discovery that comes first in the human mind. The quality of our minds leads directly to the quality of the world we make for ourselves. The technology of leisure comes from a desire to make the body comfortable. The technology of research comes from dissatisfaction with limited sight, hearing, and touch. Every desire has found a means of achieving its goal because desire and action arise at the same time. That is what we meant when we talked earlier about the "organizing power" existing inside any valid piece of knowledge.

Now we are at the point where our desire is for perfect health and longevity. What discovery is necessary for that? Our attention in the past has gone to medical technology, with brilliant results. We have staved off almost every childhood disease; we have blocked pain so that modern surgery could come into being; and we have educated whole populations to respect clean air and water, which some authorities claim has done more to extend human life than all the disease preventives put together. If our society still suffers physically, then there must be somewhere else to look. We will know when our direction is right because, as human evolution abundantly displays, whenever an advance in life is made, the desire for it and the means of achieving it are promoted by nature together.

Another observation we can easily make is that some people do manage already to live long and healthily. The psychologist Abraham Maslow devoted his career to studying such people (whom he called "self-actualized"), because he felt that a psychology based upon observing sick personalities, which is at the heart of almost all clinical psychology and psychiatry both, would not give the answer to what he wanted to know: how can man continue to grow? The answer to that question, as Maslow found out, is not futuristic or impossible. It is only necessary for the rest of us to catch up with the best of us.

The people Maslow studied were already accomplished and well rewarded by society. Their abilities to think, write, paint, compose music, treat illness, or run corporations was obviously superior. But Maslow was turning his attention to the inner man, and what he found makes all of us think about ourselves in a new way. First, he found that indeed this was a group of people who were healthier, happier, and wiser than normal. Not only did they have the attitude that life should be embraced, they also trusted themselves as creators of their own existence. As a first premise, such people believe in the goodness of the self. The remarkable thing about this belief is that it got them through many outside difficulties. For Maslow found that whenever self-actualized people faced problems outside themselves, they always turned inward for the solution. More often than not, the solution was there.

These few people — Maslow estimated that they make up less than 1 percent of the population — have discovered the psychophysiological connection on their own. More importantly, because they have such positive attitudes toward themselves, their minds and bodies work together to produce health. It is completely natural and simple for them. As Maslow put it, "What such a person wants and enjoys is apt to be just what is good for him. His spontaneous reactions are as capable, efficient and right as if they had been thought out in advance."

What is life like in general for such people? To judge by what they did, Maslow found a huge diversity in what *happened* to those he studied. However, they had in common an attitude that they were all creating something from out of themselves. The material world gave them nothing to enjoy so wonderful as the "peak experiences" that lifted them into a realm of inner freedom and creativity. These were their moments of discovery and inspiration. The people had no control over such moments, when they came and when they left. Outside their peak experiences, self-actualized people suffered and decayed and felt confused in the way everyone does. But the peak moments were enough to set them aside as quite extraordinary human beings. Besides being creative and joyous, these moments, Maslow tells us, are ones of perfect health.

So there is our clue. Once society lives up to the level of the best people it has already produced, then perfect health becomes a living reality. Healthy, creative people are our "supermen," examples of human evolution progressing in the direction of greater expansion and greater happiness. I know that "superman" is a distasteful word to many — it certainly has been put to terrible misuse in the past — but I am resorting to it intentionally because it is obvious that we cannot progress until we admit that there is a far higher plane than that of ordinary life. Significantly, Maslow discovered that weak people, those who have settled for neurosis, ill health, and unhappiness as "normal," all consistently show a fear of growing stronger. They even shun people who are demonstrably healthy, successful, loving, and wise. In a word, they are afraid to grow.

As we shall see in the course of this book, the possibility of stepping onto a higher plane is quite real for everyone. It requires no force or effort or sacrifice. It involves little more than changing our ideas about what is normal. Or, to put it in Maslow's terms, it means gaining control over peak experiences so that they are sustained every day. Being at a permanent peak is to be in the state of perfect health. As fabulous as peak experiences can sound — people speak of feeling absolute freedom, inner fulfillment, happiness devoid of doubts, an uninterrupted flow of love and creativity — the way to the peak is to follow your nose. Constant growth, if allowed to happen, will reach the peak.

The significant difference between man and superman is that man is mechanical and can do nothing about it. The actions and reactions of ordinary people are entirely predictable, and in that way they exist as no more than mechanical devices. When you apply a stimulus, you get an expected response. What Eastern thought calls "bondage of the self" is nothing mysterious; it is the habit most of us have of thinking in the same ruts all the time. If you are honest with yourself, you will notice how mechanically you behave all the time. This behavior is guided by thought patterns. Nothing outside us really changes these thoughts; they are merely triggered, and then we experience that something "made us" angry, sad, happy, or ecstatic.

We could in fact take some of the most advanced intellects of our time, people we think of as far beyond the ordinary, and prove the same thing of them. Disagree with them, and notice how upset they become. Praise them, and see how happy they are. Deride, ridicule, or criticize them, and watch them turn angry, depressed, and withdrawn. Eulogize them, glorify their achievements, and watch them swell with pride.

People who can rise above the mechanical nature of thinking do not defeat it. As Maslow found, self-actualized people are willing to accept the world and tend to feel a detachment from their own mechanical reactions to life. It was *because* they felt detached that they could love so deeply and feel true compassion and exhibit authentic wisdom. We tend to see this as contradictory, but it is not. If you are caught up in your needs, then you will utterly believe in them and make them into all you know. If you accept them as part of life and believe that they will turn out for the best, then a much larger world opens up. No one ever found a new world by worrying about it.

How, then, do we go about constantly growing in the direction of perfect health?

III

Strategies for Creating Health

The natural healing force within each one of us is the
greatest force in getting well.

— Hippocrates

21

Self-awareness

WHAT YOU PAY ATTENTION TO GROWS. If your attention is attracted to negative situations and emotions, then they will grow in your awareness. Your awareness is the composite of all the things you pay attention to. For some people, the attention is tossed about by small daily crises, bits of negativity that seem insignificant by themselves but that together are enough to keep the awareness fatigued. Psychiatrists see people in this condition every day, complaining of mild depression and free-floating anxiety. Psychiatry sometimes refers to these people as "the worried well," but they are not well. Their inner experience, their awareness, is of helplessness. They never quite come to a crisis, yet they never adequately focus their energies either.

When the attention finds something meaningful to focus on, a significant goal, it takes a step closer to creating health. A goal gives people something to live for — a project, a profession, a family — and the body responds with vitality. This sort of awareness replenishes energy. The goal-oriented person wakes up each morning ready to devote himself to the task at hand. However, if the project fails or the age of retirement arrives or a family member dies suddenly, such people are often propelled into depression or illness. Their intense concentration on a goal puts them in a precarious position in the long run, because their awareness runs in one narrow channel. The river of life will not run in just one channel.

The highest state of attention goes beyond goals. It is not excited by circumstances or pulled about by daily crises. The inner landscape is serene and, above all, quiet. As much attention has been paid to rest as to activity. The awareness is therefore balanced, vital, and comprehensive. We perceive such people as deeply quiet and very understanding about life. Being paid attention to by them makes us relax. The calmness they breathe is very close to wisdom. It is the true foundation for creating health. It is called self-awareness.

Anyone who has reached self-awareness, even intermittently, or who has spent time around a self-aware person knows that this quality cannot be valued too highly. The power of force and the power of money are trivial beside the power of self-knowledge. It produces positive attitudes all the time, not by working for them, but by allowing life to deliver them. Resisting or opposing our negative thoughts is just another form of paying attention to them. What we pay attention to grows. Here is the Indian thinker Krishnamurti on the futility of struggling with our negative thought patterns:

> It is no good trying to polish stupidity, trying to become clever. First I must know that I am stupid, that I am dull. The very awareness of my dullness is to be free of my dullness, to say, "I am a fool," not verbally, but actually say, "Well, I am a fool," then you are already watchful; you are no longer a fool. But if you resist what you are, then your dullness becomes more and more. In the world the apogee of intellect is to be very clever, very smart, very complex, very erudite, but erudition has nothing to do with intelligence. To see things as they are, in ourselves, without bringing about conflict in perceiving what we are, needs the tremendous simplicity of intelligence.

Krishnamurti is telling us that when attention is innocent, free from conditioning, it is most powerful. Only self-awareness knows this. The so-called tender emotions spring from the source of life; therefore, they are incredibly powerful. Inner awareness creates health because it is vital. We only have to look at the radiance of a new mother or the play of a happy child to see this life-enhancing state. The attention is allowing life to flow through it, and the result must be healthy.

Our mechanical nature keeps us inattentive. Our true nature, our selves, our intelligence, cannot help us if we do not pay attention to it. What you do not pay attention to will not grow. When attention is properly attuned — without excitement, without effort — then self-awareness simply happens. It opens the channel through which the brain can consistently bring health to the body. A simple kind of intelligence makes itself felt everywhere in the physiology without fuss. In the presence of quiet attention, there are no such things as anger, fear, suspicion, greed, guilt, intolerance, anxiety, or depression. They disappear like paper tigers.

But they are real tigers until they do disappear. As long as we pay attention to them, they will grow. Still, it is eminently healthy to know in advance, before we seriously engage in techniques of gaining self-awareness, that it is useless to fight against what is negative in ourselves. All strategies for creating health start here.

22

Living in the Present

Health is the only thing that makes you feel that now is the
best time of the year.

— Franklin Adams

Yesterday is but a dream, tomorrow is but a vision. But
today well lived makes every yesterday a dream of happiness and every tomorrow a vision of hope. Look well,
therefore, to this day.

— Sanskrit proverb

HAVE YOU EVER HEARD someone say, "Worry causes aging"?
There is tremendous truth to it. Everybody has seen people "turn
gray overnight" when they underwent a financial or emotional
crisis. What exactly is this pattern of thoughts we call worry? It
seems to have a powerful ability to poison many hours of our existence; we could even say that worry causes aging because it
speeds up time. Worry is obviously a certain habit of thought. It is
fretting about something that has already happened in the past or
about something that we fear will happen in the future. Worry
does not deal in the present.

Let us look first at the past. No one has discovered a means of
altering the past. Once a thing has occurred, there is no way to
change it. It is indelibly and irrevocably recorded; time has carried
it off beyond anyone's efforts to make improvements. Dwelling on
past mistakes or injuries is unproductive. It is also harmful, because it releases into your system all kinds of toxic substances that
raise blood pressure and strain the heart. The strategy that dis-
arms worry is to recognize past mistakes for what they are, learn

from them, and then leave them in their permanent home, the past. Devoting one's attention to the present requires a healthy realization that the past is gone forever. Worry is the psychological refusal to face this. What makes it a seemingly inevitable part of living is that mistakes, injuries, grudges, and acts of injustice leave an impression on the mind and seep into the physiology through the psychophysiological connection.

The second kind of worry is fixated on the future. It is caught up in avoiding pain by futilely trying to control the future. A medical colleague of mine, an internist, furnished me with a compelling example of this style of thought. He had been treating a woman for the last twenty years, and over that period she visited him twice a year for a complete physical. Whenever she came, she showed a great concern to him about having cancer. Although she displayed no symptoms of the disease at all, she would concoct a series of complaints that forced the internist to run a battery of tests merely to reassure her that she did not have cancer.

This scenario repeated itself year in and year out. Each time, the internist did his best to reassure his patient that she was free of cancer, and each time she left him asking, "Are you sure?" On the last occasion, however, her physician ran his tests and had grim news. He confronted the woman with a confirmed diagnosis of cancer. To which, raising herself up in a kind of triumph, she replied, "I told you so! I have been telling you so for the last twenty years!"

In her worrying, this woman vividly imagined a disease she greatly feared, and what she paid attention to grew. Awareness itself has a way of altering events. Our subconscious mind quite automatically can turn things we vividly imagine into reality. People who worry have convinced themselves that worry is somehow the right *style* of thought for making something bad not happen. In reality, however, attention is attention. If we vividly imagine something we do not want to happen, it is almost certainly bound to happen. Perhaps something "just as bad" happens; it amounts to the same thing. If we must imagine the future at all, it needs to be an imagination of joyful, happy, positive things.

Healthy people, however, live neither in the past nor in the future. They live in the present, in the *now,* which gives the now a flavor of eternity because no shadows fall across it. Worry does not occur in the present. When attention is paid to the present moment, it grows in its own fullness. When a life is spent in ever-successive moments of now, then time is not the psychological enemy of man. The mischief of worry is defeated by appreciation for what life has to give today.

23

Ego Gratification

HARD AS IT IS to believe, I have several patients who enjoy being sick. In fact, I have some who become happier as they become sicker. One of these patients, who is chronically ill with a condition of the intestines called ulcerative colitis, goes through cycles when she becomes acutely sick, at times dangerously so. During the periods when she is chronically sick — that is, most of the time — she spends long visits to my office complaining about how miserable she feels, how she cannot do this or that, and how her one wish is just to die.

During those episodes when she is acutely and dangerously sick, however, she displays the most quiet, relaxed, and at times quite exasperatingly carefree attitude. She may be bleeding profusely from her lower intestine, and her blood count may show profound anemia, but she insists that she feels absolutely normal. Despite protestations from her family and entreaties from me, she refuses to go into the hospital, maintaining that there is nothing to worry about, she will get better. When she is chronically sick, she constantly seeks attention. When acutely sick, or even moribund, she enjoys the gratification of not having to seek attention at all — she gets it automatically. The whole illness revolves around the state of her ego and its need to feel important and attract the attention it deserves.

Ego gratification is a basic human need. The lack of it leads to imbalance, sometimes derangement, in the emotions and the physiology. This poor woman I was treating became sick to gratify her ego. Her extremely risky and unhealthy approach to ego gratification created tremendous strain on her system. This condition is the opposite of what Abraham Maslow described when he said that really healthy personalities need and enjoy what turns out to be good for them.

As a physician, I see patients every day whose maladies grow worse or better according to the patient's ego needs. In other words, the onset of disease processes is intimately connected to a deficiency of ego gratification. What are these deficiencies? They are quite common things: lack of feeling important, lack of appreciation, lack of approval and encouragement, lack of love.

Your ego feeds on appreciation, encouragement, and love. We find it easier to face vitamin or mineral deficiency in the body than ego deficiencies, which are actually more significant for most people. When any basic human need goes unfulfilled, it can lead to disastrous results, to disease and infirmity. If we look around, we readily observe that happy and healthy people seem to have an abundance of love, appreciation, praise, and importance. One belief that works against giving this appreciation in our society is the idea that people should not be praised or made to feel important, for this is said to give them a sense of false superiority or self-satisfaction. Psychology has repeatedly shown that this attitude is wrong. Praise, love, and appreciation lead to a balanced and sane sense of inner worth. Without them, the ego does not know where to stand. It is continually swinging between exaggerated feelings of worthlessness and exaggerated fantasies of self-importance.

Unhappy, unhealthy people, who hunger most for attention, never seem to get it. A great deal of clinical attention has gone into analyzing this and trying to correct it. I think that the answer is simple and the way out direct. In one of its best-known formulations, the technique for ego gratification is this: "Do unto others as you would have them do unto you." If you want praise, praise others. If you feel insufficiently appreciated, direct more appreciation to people around you. If you crave love, then innocently allow yourself to be loving. If you want importance, make other people feel important, and do it sincerely.

There is nothing new about this technique. Every tradition of wisdom has included some version of "for as you sow, so shall you reap." The problem of course is that knowing about this and acting upon it are two different things. The schools of "positive thinking" have sprung up so that people can learn to employ the enormous power of giving in order to receive. For a few individuals, positive thinking is easy to slip into and therefore works. But the mind is much deeper than superficial thoughts, or even thoughts about thoughts. At its deepest level, the mind is *already* reaping what it sows. Every thought is being automatically translated into a style of physiology. If the cooperation of mind and body is harmonious, then the flow of life itself will bring with it a full appreciation of life. Ego gratification will come about as one of the natural gifts of health.

For a far greater number of people, the obstacles to ego gratification are quite real. They are experienced as doubt, worry, guilt, denial of pleasure, and preoccupation with the self. These are the contents of a bad conscience. Under their spell, the ego can gratify itself only through devious routes. In that sense, all neurosis and self-inflicted disease is like a detour. In order for the straight road to become apparent, there must be self-awareness.

24

The Importance of Job Satisfaction

Work should be performed in the spirit of worship.

— Napoleon Hill

Various are our acts, various are the occupations of men. The carpenter desires timber, the physician disease, the Brahman a worshipper who offers soma.

— Rig Veda

NUMEROUS STUDIES at various medical centers have agreed on the fact that people live longer, healthier lives if they are satisfied with their jobs. We spend one-third of our lives practicing our chosen vocation. If we are unhappy at work, it is bound to carry over into the hours after work. It is bound to make us unhappy all the time and therefore prone to ill health and physical deterioration.

Time after time I see patients in my office whose medical problems I can directly relate to their dissatisfaction with work. They just hate what they are doing and spend their working hours filled with hostility, resentment, and frustration, accomplishing little on the job or in life. After they come home, they find it less and less easy to recover from their work moods, and they vent their resentment through smoking, drinking, and overeating. Their sleep is disturbed by incessant worry over work and dissatisfaction with what they get out of work. I see them with haggard, tired expressions on their faces, complaining of symptoms such as migraine, heart palpitations, insomnia, obesity, hypertension, and anxiety. They look and feel biologically older than their chronological age.

My clinical observation over the years leads me to believe that people who are unhappy with their jobs actually suffer from serious ailments more frequently than people who work hard and are happy at what they do. There is some truth to being "too busy to get sick." Idleness is therefore not the answer, for I observe that people recently laid off from work or generally unemployed have a greater incidence of complaints affecting every bodily system. Their bodies are suffering the same kind of atrophy that nature shows everywhere when something grows useless. In the scheme of things, what is useless soon dies out. Nature, and this includes our inner nature, has no room for what is useless. It promotes health only in those things that contribute to growth and increased development. To progress is to survive.

Physiotherapists and exercise physiologists are well aware of a phenomenon called disuse atrophy. This is the wasting away of a limb or organ that is not being used. Once the limb is made useful and functioning again, the process is reversed. Blood begins to flow in the part that was turning lifeless, and the more function is restored, the stronger and more powerful that part of the body becomes. Activity, usefulness, and progress by themselves are great secrets of longevity and health. Emerson put it beautifully when he said, "People do not grow old; when they cease to grow, they become old."

Feel and be useful. Contribute to the growth of the life you are part of. People who hear this advice often conclude that they are in the wrong profession; this may be so. But generally it is their negative attitude that has poisoned any opportunity for job satisfaction. Every job serves some useful purpose, for there is always someone who can use it for his own evolution and growth. The social usefulness of work was its traditional source of importance, and so jobs came into existence because they filled concrete needs. But evolution has clearly shifted the emphasis to personal growth in our century; therefore, people demand personal satisfaction with their work, not because they are more selfish than older generations, but because they quite accurately perceive that the primary usefulness of work is to the self.

People who feel useful do not deteriorate or get unhealthy. Rooted in satisfaction with themselves, they stand ready to make the collective work prosper. However, the pyramid of jobs obviously includes far more routine jobs at the bottom than creative ones at the top. It is the grind of routine that my patients suffer from when they bring their symptoms to me. The first thing to say is that jobs at the top do tend to go to healthier people, those who are naturally able to achieve more, but I think that their positive attitudes came first and created the possibilities for promotion. Any job, routine or not, involves repetition and discipline. The person who lacks inner awareness inevitably and quickly comes to the point where the repetitiveness of his work brings on boredom and fatigue. From that all the later symptoms grow.

The person who is secure in himself finds creative solutions to routine work. He is not in the habit of noticing what is boring, tiring, or repetitive. Such people have the courage in the first place to find jobs that they like. They do not worry about financial security when their happiness is at stake. Once they do find a job that satisfies them, they keep at it without thought of retirement. This is because what life has to offer them is already found at work: growth, progress, and prosperity. If you are desperate for leisure, then your work is killing you. If you cannot wait for retirement, then you are retired already, so far as happiness on the job is concerned.

As a physician I cannot help my patients by getting better jobs for them or by making them like the jobs they already have. I can only temporarily help them by treating their symptoms. But by leading them to a healthy, spontaneous awareness of the self, I can point out where the true solution lies.

25

Channeling the Unconscious Mind —
The Force of Habit

EVERY IMPULSE OF INTELLIGENCE needs a channel to follow. When we speak of growing in awareness, we have to be talking about new channels for intelligence, otherwise, self-awareness would be no more than an amorphous mood. A consciously created channel for intelligence is called a habit. Ordinarily we tend to think of habits as rather drab parts of the daily routine — the same toothbrush, the same orange juice, the same wife. But every type of skill or talent depends upon habit. Lift the hand to drive a nail, and that desire, translated via a fixed channel into a physical action, could turn into the dexterity of a master carpenter. Lay your index finger on the key for middle C on a piano, and you are doing what a virtuoso habituated himself to do years ago and still does today through the force of habit.

The force of habit is practically impossible to stop once its channel has been opened. The conscious mind may tell itself that it can control everyday habits — lose weight when it wants to, quit smoking, accept new beliefs and think unknown thoughts — but the force of habit is like a tidal wave and the conscious mind its precariously perched rider. Habit cares very little, for instance, whether we think of it as good or bad. We have all heard the cry of the chain smoker, "I didn't even want that cigarette," and the dieter's "I didn't even feel hungry when I ate that pie." In order to see why habit is so strong, we have to look a little closer at the nature of the mind.

Psychologists usually divide the mind into conscious and unconscious. By conscious mind, which is said to account for no more than 10 percent of brain function, we generally mean those thoughts that are under our conscious control or that we have awareness of as ideas. The unconscious mind, more than 90 percent of the total, is a much shaggier beast and not too well understood; it is, after all, not conscious. Freud named it the *id,* which is simply Latin for "it." But the unconscious yields up many of its mysteries when we look to our knowledge about brain physiology, none of which was available to Freud in his lifetime.

Brain physiologists tell us that different parts of the brain are responsible for specific functions, and when those parts are activated, the functions occur. Only a small number of these functions (specifically, the abstract thinking and so-called higher activity of the cerebral cortex) seem to be in our conscious awareness. But current brain research informs us that any one thought can activate many parts of the brain at once. A single thought, therefore, is not like a blip on a mental screen; it is much more like a newspaper photo made up of thousands of dots arranged in a precise pattern to make one image.

With this in mind, we see that the unconscious and conscious parts of the mind are not separate. The mind has no divisions or rigid compartments; we simply create them in order to talk about the mind. At any one time, your *whole* brain is working, but your awareness or attention only brings to the surface those aspects of the whole that make up your thought or emotion or inspiration of the moment. In order to have any thought, however, you must set up channels that literally run through the entire body. That is what we meant when we spoke earlier of the "pathways" that convert thoughts to physical responses via the psychophysiological connection. When these channels are complete and free of stress, then there is health. When they are obstructed or wrongly formed, then there is ill health. It is all a matter of giving intelligence the right paths to follow; therefore, it is largely a matter of habit.

Every habit is a cooperative venture between body and mind. Generally speaking, the mind leads the venture and the body follows as a silent partner. This works very well when the habit is something suitable like swinging a tennis racket or playing the violin. The tremendous skill that the body shows in sports or musical performance is made possible by the simple fact that the athlete or musician does not have to think about what he is doing. His faintest intention is translated into incredibly coordinated responses of mind and body. He is taking supreme advantage of mind-body coordination thanks to the force of habit.

But as we saw when we discussed disease symptoms, the mechanical nature of habit can work for ill. If the mind has a faint intention to gain gratification, but the channels automatically set up for that include smoking, drinking, or overeating, then the force of habit will carry the body toward disease. The partnership of mind and body is like a balloon: if you squeeze it in one place, it always bulges out somewhere else. In a bad habit, the body gives way as much as it can to accommodate the mind's desire, for example, allowing blood pressure to rise, stress hormones to activate improperly the fight-or-flight response, and heartbeat to increase, but in time the stressed parts of the body grow to fit the bulge, and then there is no more flexibility left. The outcome is chronic high blood pressure, an exhausted hormone system, and a strained heart.

Fortunately, there is no limit to the number of new channels that intelligence is willing to follow. When we say that the potential of the human mind — of *your* mind — is infinite, this flexibility of intelligence is the practical reality that makes such a claim valid. Any single habit involves the whole central nervous system's communicating billions of impulses to the whole body. Our mind may be conscious only of swinging a tennis racket, but the changes in biochemistry at the level of the cell membranes alone that carry out this action would require an enormous computer to analyze, not to mention the astounding complexity involved as intelligence activates hormones, enzymes, muscle reactions, and the brain parts needed for balance, focused eyesight, strategic thinking, and so on. Any response that includes billions of changes also leads to billions upon billions of new combinations from the same elements — and that gives intelligence a world of new channels to play in.

If we want to create health, starting this moment, then we have to start channeling the unconscious mind through habit. In my experience, any approach to new habits should follow these guidelines: the habit should be acquired effortlessly over a period of time, it should be guided by positive thoughts, and it should be consciously repeated, but always in a good frame of mind, never forced in as the enemy of a bad habit. Cultivated in this way, new habits condition the whole mind-body system to create health and happiness automatically. I am again reminded of those two sentences from Abraham Maslow about very healthy, creative people: "What such a person wants and enjoys is apt to be just what is good for him. His spontaneous reactions are as capable, efficient and right as if they had been thought out in advance." It sounds too good to be true, but it is just habit at work.

All that is needed is the awareness that the unconscious mind can be changed in its routine, and then one simply changes it. People who have been unhappy all their lives can become happy simply by realizing that the source of change is inside themselves. The responsibility for all illness and all cure resides with us. The unconscious can be refined and rechanneled through suggestion, repetition, and above all attention. It is attention, or awareness, that touches the sleeping powers of mind and makes them vital again. Do not fret too much over "how it all happens" — that is just an old mindset saying, "It won't happen, it can't." The smallest shift in attention can change the world you perceive and the body you live with. When you buy a rose, you also buy its thorns. If you notice the rose, you have an experience of beauty; if you notice the thorns, you have an experience of pain.

Healthy habits, then, cannot be overvalued as forces for health. Let me give you a start. At the Weimar Institute in California, I saw a poster that read, "New Start — God's Natural Remedies," which turned out to be a coded message about creating health:

N Nutrition
E Exercise
W Water

S Sunshine
T Temperance
A Air
R Rest
T Trust in God and Control of One's Thought Processes

Most of these elements we have already touched upon, and most of the others simply remind us that a natural life, when all is said and done, really will achieve astonishing results that medicine cannot rival. Clean air and water, nutritious food, moderate activity, a little walk in the sunshine, and a good night's sleep: the key here is habit. These are all powerful preventives of ill health if you make them habits. Occasional good habits are no habits at all. The point is to allow creative intelligence, or the mind-body connection, to work *automatically*. If you have to think about "being good," then your body is not accustomed to health, and in fact your occasional "good" can be quite harmful.

As medical experience attests, the person who only golfs on Sunday or works outside when he has to shovel snow off the driveway is making himself susceptible to muscle strain and heart failure. The most dangerous skin cancers, called melanomas, are most likely to happen not to people who work in the sun all the time or who stay indoors all the time but to people who get severely blistered once a year on their vacations. Even doing this as a child and never again is capable of triggering the abnormal mind-body responses that wind up years later as malignancy. So approach habits gradually but consistently and do not cultivate any but the ones you actually like.

Two habits on the list call for a little comment. *Temperance* is a word that is easy to misunderstand, but it simply means not doing anything to excess. This is very important, not for moral reasons, but because body mechanisms work within limits, and moderation in eating, rest, work, and exercise respects those limits. Habit will channel an enormous organizing power from the unconscious mind, but only if the mind-body connection is allowed to flow smoothly. Billions of things are happening every time you think a thought or move a finger, but in reality only one thing is happening — intelligence is flowing. Doing anything to excess creates stress, which we have already defined as "whatever blocks the flow of creative intelligence."

"Trust in God and Control of One's Thought Processes" is not given here by me as a religious dictum. I am pointing out in every chapter the evidence for an infinite intelligence that permeates nature and expresses itself through our minds and bodies. It alone brings perfect health; its simple, unobstructed flow is the only "control" that can mastermind the myriad processes of life. The only attitude that we can meaningfully have toward it is trust.

26

Diet and Destiny

Food is Brahman.

— Rig Veda

From food are born all creatures, which live upon food and after death return to food. Food is the chief of all things. It is therefore said to be medicine for all diseases of the body. Those who worship food as Brahman gain all material objects. From food are born all beings, which being born, grow by food. All beings feed upon food, and when they die, food feeds upon them.

— Taittiraya Upanishad

A LIFE BEGINS as desire. Impulses of intelligence that we call love and desire are transformed through our parents into the fusion of minute amounts of genetic material that we call an embryo. So we are conceived out of love and desire, and start life as genetic material. However minute, the DNA that composes this genetic material contains within it the entire blueprint of our destiny. The raw material of DNA is sugar and a complex chemical called nucleic acid. The complexity of nucleic acid is enough, when built up into DNA, to encode the complete intelligence that out of love and desire our parents bestowed upon the first conceived cell.

We are nurtured by the sum total of love, desire, and intelligence, all infused into one raw material whose common name is — food. Food transformed, given consciousness, is us. If we want a potato or a grain of buckwheat to become as conscious as we ourselves are, we eat it. The intelligence that permeates every cell of the body then sets to work on that bit of food. Nothing dramatic really happens to it. The chemical constituents of its nutrients are simply shifted so that they can enter our cells. The material of food becomes every part of us — eyes, hair, brain, bowel. Here is creation, and the act of eating and assimilating food involves the infinite intelligence of the universe playing itself out through this specific act of creation. Nature began the universe by creating itself in the form of titanic explosions of mass-energy that led to unimaginably huge galaxies and nebulae. But when it evolved sufficiently to create something really complex, nature learned to eat.

Consider this: I drink a glass of orange juice. Every single cell in my body (which contains billions and billions of cells) encounters every molecule of glucose from that juice. Every cell in my body partakes of the share of the orange juice it needs, and out of simple need it converts the juice into itself. The intricacies of what the cell has done, insofar as science now understands it, are enough to fill large spaces in the libraries of the world. When you are aware of the complexity and at the same time of the simplicity, innocence, and elegance with which the organizing power of intelligence transforms food into human beings and all creatures of the earth, then you are ready to participate in your destiny. You can sit down and eat.

People who do not feel sufficient respect for eating are showing no awareness of the flow of organizing power that it represents. Eating indiscriminately or eating unconsciously, eating on the run, habitually overeating or not eating at all — these are all violations of natural law, that is, of the biological processes that must work in their preordained channels in order for food to be converted into us. Innumerable disorders are linked to diet and eating habits. For example, it is estimated that more than 90 percent of the cases of gastrointestinal cancer, including major killers like cancer of the colon, are directly related to nutrition. The high blood pressure, elevated blood cholesterol, and serious heart disease that is epidemic in Western societies, not to mention diabetes, hypoglycemia, ulcers, and gouty arthritis, demonstrate obvious connections to bad eating habits and wrong food.

I do not believe that it is necessary for us to become nutritionists in order to eat right. In fact, I want to give very little detailed dietary advice in this book just to point up the more important truth: the intelligence of our bodies knows what is good for it. Once that intelligence is channeled through correct habits — and this involves making conscious decisions at the beginning — then eating problems and the risks of a wrong diet disappear.

An overweight person may disagree at this point, protesting that his body cannot seem to help itself when confronted with food. But consider this: if you gain ten pounds a year, which in a few years would make you overweight and grossly obese in a decade, you are still overeating by only an average of less than one hundred calories a day. That amounts to little more than a tablespoon of oil, a third of a candy bar, or half a handful of peanuts. In other words, even chronic, "uncontrollable" weight gain involves a tiny adjustment in the body's idea of what is the right amount to eat. By the same logic, a tiny adjustment in the opposite direction will bring the weight down. This adjustment must begin in the mind, starting with an intention to respect the body's intelligence.

We are constantly barraged on all sides by diet information. Some of it serves the interests of producers who have food to sell, some is pushed by medical interests that want to reverse the trends of disease, and there is much else besides. All of it is irrelevant once the cells of your body begin to get through to your brain information about what they want: a moderate amount of nutrients supplied in variety at regular times of the day. New habits that move in this direction are worth more than any advice from a diet authority.

It is time to reflect for a moment: how reasonable is our obsession with vitamins, minerals, proteins, and the rest of our diet? The amount of information we store in our brains about nutrition seems to me irrelevant to health as a natural state of the body. How likely is it that birds in the forest suffer from vitamin D deficiency? Is there a single living species on earth besides man that regulates its life according to "recommended daily allowances" of any nutrient? Nutritional authorities understand and have repeatedly stated that our knowledge of nutrients is sketchy at best.

Most of this information was obtained by starving animals of various nutrients until they showed a certain deficiency disease. Much of the rest came from observing people who had already contracted deficiency diseases. So what is known depends far too much on studying abnormal states of physiology. Yet it is also well known that each cell of the body has a precise ability to select from the diet exactly what it needs in order to grow. That is why all premodern societies got enough vitamin C to stave off scurvy, even though they consciously knew nothing whatever about vitamin C and did not drink orange juice every morning.

Nature has not left us worse off than birds and reptiles and other mammals. It is true that we have incorporated into ourselves some wrong habits over the years that now obscure our innate intelligence, but intelligence cannot actually be eradicated. Our instincts for proper nourishment have been dulled in part by listening to people who tell us what to eat, what is supposed to taste good, what is good for us, and what is not good for us. The best advice I have heard in this regard came from Dr. Wayne Dyer, who said, "First, be a good animal." When we come to the last part of the book, I will talk about a means of restoring automatic and correct behavior to all parts of the psychophysiological system, which is called "spontaneous right action."

For the moment, recognizing that most people want perfect health but are far from knowing how to activate their inner intelligence, I want to give a few guidelines about eating. They come from my own observation and are not the official recommendations of scientific medicine at large. There are other physicians, however, who would absolutely agree with me. What all the points that follow have in common is this: they gently but continuously prompt your body and mind to join together in a flow of intelligence. As in other aspects of health, once that flow is set up, nothing else is necessary but to enjoy your life.

1. Pay attention to eating
2. Pause momentarily before eating and sit in silence — or say grace — so that the awareness begins the meal quietly

3. Eat when you are hungry, and do not eat when you are not hungry
4. Do not sit down to eat if you are upset — your body is better off without food until you feel better
5. Take time to eat, chewing food well and slowly
6. Appreciate the company and compliment the cook
7. Avoid eating in any company that makes you feel less than agreeable, but eat with congenial company, friends and family, when you can

In our times, some of this advice may look strange. Our times are the exception, however. Every culture has lived by these customs, for that is what they are, and has found in them the solid comfort of a healthy life. Man's everyday attitude toward food has been thankfulness. In his moments of deepest reflection, this attitude turns to reverence. Good food, abundantly provided, and taken with appreciativeness, is a sign that man welcomes his ties with nature, and nature has responded by nourishing him well.

The Case for Vegetarianism

Along with many other physicians, I am convinced that a vegetarian diet is the best one for health. A vegetarian is one who lives wholly or primarily on a diet without meat. Although some vegetarians refrain from eating meat because they abhor the idea of slaughtering animals, this approach does not enter into the argument here. Also, if your diet comes to include eggs, chicken, and fish in small amounts, I think that you will gain the same health benefits that strict vegetarians do. Most human societies have subsisted on nearly vegetarian diets throughout history, so in a sense it is a norm and not a special "dietary practice." We tend to rationalize that Europeans lived on cabbage and millet for centuries out of poverty, or that Asians subsist on rice and vegetables today because of overpopulation.

The truth is that the human physiology sustains health best

when its intake of meat fat and proteins is small or nonexistent. The American Dietetic Association, in a pamphlet titled *The Vegetarian Approach to Eating,* observes that "a growing body of scientific evidence supports a positive relationship between the consumption of a plant-based diet and the prevention of certain diseases." The following diseases have been definitely linked to our ordinary diet that is high in meat and animal fats:

1. *Coronary artery disease:* Its exact cause is unknown, but a growing mass of evidence suggests that coronary artery disease, the number one killer in our society, is a chronic, degenerative disorder related to diet. Saturated fats and cholesterol-rich foods have definitely been linked to hardening of the arteries (atherosclerosis), which is the condition that leads to coronary artery disease.

Saturated fats and cholesterol come to us primarily in meat, cheese, eggs, and butter. When the diet shifts to foods derived from plants, there is a definite decrease in the levels of cholesterol in the blood. Coronary artery disease is known to be from 30 percent to 50 percent less common among long-term vegetarians such as Seventh-Day Adventists, who advocate vegetarianism as part of their religious beliefs. These people also tend to have other good habits, such as not smoking, but nonvegetarian Seventh-Day Adventists who were studied showed a death rate from heart attacks three times greater than that of vegetarians of the sect who were the same age.

2. *Cancer:* I have already covered the diet-cancer connection in the first part of this book, but I will repeat here that colon and breast cancer are linked to high intake of fats and cholesterol and that diets low in plant-derived fiber are implicated in several cancers of the digestive tract. All responsible agencies, including the American Cancer Society, now recommend lowering the intake of meat in order to lower the risk of cancer.

3. *Obesity:* The popular idea that eating a diet full of bread, potatoes, rice, beans, pasta, and other staples of the vegetarian diet makes you fat is not founded on facts. As we have already seen, obesity is linked to numerous health risks and to almost every

major disease. Studies show consistently that Americans who eat meat weigh more than those who do not.

4. *Dental caries:* Caries of the teeth, commonly called cavities, occur less frequently among vegetarians than among meat eaters.

5. *Osteoporosis:* This disorder is a thinning of the bones and loss of bone mass that seriously affects many women past the age of menopause, leading to spinal problems and frequent, slow-to-heal fractures as they grow to old age. Although meat is a good source of bone calcium (so are low-fat dairy products, fish, beans, and leafy green vegetables), studies indicate that a high-protein diet eaten over a long period of time leads to calcium and bone loss.

As these facts are assimilated by the mainstream of the American population, vegetarian diets will become more common; they are already common enough that even athletes, who traditionally have eaten lots of red meat at the training table, are seeing the value of eating carbohydrates for energy instead. (The classic study on this, conducted decades ago at Yale, showed that no athlete who ate meat could sustain the same endurance levels as the lowest-ranked vegetarian in the tests.) A steady stream of energy from whole grains and other complete-carbohydrate foods is much better for the system in general than spurts of energy from sugar (or alcohol), and the digestive system has an easier time working on such foods than on fats and animal proteins. In any event, statistics on the baby boom generation, which is now between thirty and forty years old, indicate that smoking, drinking, and heavy consumption of meat have declined. We can expect the epidemic of lifestyle diseases to drop dramatically.

For those who want to make a shift in the direction of vegetarianism, I can provide guidelines that are generally agreed upon. (You might also look at the remarks on diet in chapter 4 on cancer and chapter 6 on obesity — these chapters cover the topic of disease prevention through nutrition.)

1. Do not change your diet suddenly and drastically. Make gradual changes, preferably at moments when you feel relaxed, expansive, and unpressured.

2. Begin by favoring fish and poultry over red meat, and eat smaller portions of them if that seems called for.

3. Eat real cooking, not penitential bowls of beans, rice, or boiled vegetables. Almost all the Asian cuisines are based on vegetables and rice, with small portions of meat. Italian pasta dishes are also low in meat protein or even entirely vegetarian.

4. Whenever you have a choice, choose whole-grain breads, muffins, and cereals in place of refined white flour. Whole grains provide complete protein for the body in any combination with nuts, legumes (beans or lentils), or seeds. Any vegetarian meal with either milk or tofu as part of it is bound to contain complete protein too.

General Recommendations

Although quite a few books of sound nutritional advice are on the market, I have seen none that tells us how to cultivate the body's flow of intelligence so that in time it tells us automatically what we should eat. So I will try to give suggestions in that direction, with the caution that they are based upon my own observations and medical reading, not on a body of current research. In part IV of this book I talk about approaching creative intelligence through the mind, which is ultimately the approach that makes perfect health a practical reality in all aspects of life. However, the current wave of interest in diet prompts me to make the following points:

1. The body wants a moderate amount of food containing various nutrients at regular times in the day. If you are already providing this (and do not smoke or drink), then you are doing the main things that allow the body to balance its metabolism and digestion. The body loves habit. Eat at about the same time every day, eat about the same amounts every day, and eat a little bit of everything.

2. When the body's intelligence is fully working, then your taste buds are an excellent guide to what you should be eating. What is good for you should be exactly what you like. Most of us

are misled by our palate because we stimulate it in the wrong way or we overstimulate it. In order to restore the taste buds, it is helpful to

- reduce the amount of salt that you add to your food and do not eat salty snacks before meals
- stop stimulating the palate with alcohol before meals and do not drink at all if that is possible
- drink tepid, not cold, water to cleanse the palate as you eat
- move in the direction of appreciating the natural taste of food by including all the tastes in every meal, that is, things that are sweet, sour, bitter, and salty.

3. If strong food cravings are a problem, do not try to tackle them head on. They represent deeply ingrained habits or strong but misguided messages from your physiology. Simply eat other foods that are part of a balanced diet. When a craving for sweets or salt or another favorite taste strikes, try eating half of what you crave, but do not pressure yourself.

4. Learn how to tell when you have eaten enough. The body has a signal for this, called the satiety response. It operates quite naturally if the diet has lots of grains, bulky foods, and liquid in it, for these quickly fill you up. A diet high in fat, salt, and sugar tends to throw this response off, however. An easy way to cultivate the satiety response is to drink water with your meal and eat bread before you start on the meal itself. (In one study, students told to eat two slices of whole-wheat bread at the start of every meal showed consistent weight loss in a few months. This is a good example of effortless dieting.)

5. Take your largest meal at lunch and eat only two-thirds of what fills you up. These two habits help to develop actual hunger, which is the body's only valid signal of when to eat. Heavy eating at night strains the system and promotes irregular digestion.

6. Accustom yourself to nothing but fresh food. I have saved this point for last because I hope it will stick in your mind. Nature intended us to eat fresh, natural foods. Although our bodies can adjust to canned or frozen food, leftovers and processed food, adulterated and "junk" food, eating these is not the way to attain

perfect health. Eating fresh food, freshly cooked at every meal, is everyone's correct diet. If you do not like to cook, then go to a restaurant for a wholesome, balanced, cooked-to-order lunch, eat it at a comfortable pace, and then have a sandwich and milk for dinner. If you breakfast only on orange juice, coffee, and a doughnut, then change to oatmeal, whole-wheat toast, and milk, or to whatever variation of the traditional hot American breakfast you enjoy. It will quickly help to restore a physiology that experiences energy slumps during the day.

27

Rhythms, Rest, and Activity

When an electron vibrates, the universe shakes.

— Sir Arthur Eddington

The same stream of life that runs through my veins
night and day, runs through the world and dances in
rhythmic measure.

— Rabindranath Tagore

NATURE FUNCTIONS IN CYCLES of rest and activity. We live in a
pulsating universe, and its pulsations are reflected in every level of
existence. The wave nature of light, the immensely long life cycles
of stars, the ebb and flow of the earth's seas, and the breathing of
living things are all variations of activity alternating with rest. An
ancient Vedic text from India declares that the universe is the
macrocosm and man the microcosm. Our cells pulse in a rhythm
whose timekeeper is the universe as a whole. The flow of intelligence that regulates mind and body in us attends to its own cycles
and functions best when these cycles are closely heeded.

Contemporary science has yet to agree on how universal
rhythms and biological rhythms exactly interact, but simple observation brings into view four natural cycles that contribute their
rhythms to ours. They are: (1) the rotation of the earth on its axis,
which creates the cycle of day and night; (2) the orbiting of the
earth around the sun, which creates the cycle of the seasons; (3)
the motion of the moon around the earth, observed as phases of
the moon, which creates the cycle of the lunar month; and (4) the

shifting gravitational forces of earth, moon, and sun throughout the year, observed in the rise and fall of the tides.

In the past few centuries, our observation of these rhythms has directed itself outward, so people now tend to think of them as facts of astronomy. However, every living thing is biologically programmed through its genes to respond to these rhythms, including humans. The birds do not migrate because they observe the seasons, nor do fruits ripen or seeds sprout or bears hibernate because they keep a lookout. Nature's rhythms are in them, and their intelligence is therefore always moving in cycles. The days and seasons of the year also profoundly affect human beings. The vast majority of people outside cities still wake and sleep, reap and sow, work and rest, grow and decline according to rhythms set by nature, not by humans.

Since these rhythms are not outside ourselves, we do not have to conjure them at the level of thought. But it is important to respect them and not strain our physiology to oppose them. Medical research is discovering that the balance of fluid in the cells and of electrolytes in the blood plasma appears to fluctuate with lunar phases; this balance is following the tides of the ocean. The heartbeat sets up its constant wave patterns in the blood stream; the various brain wave patterns are so complicated that research is just beginning to comprehend their motions, what one pioneer investigator, J. Lhermitte, called "this winged and fleeting thing that is mind." The body's hormones are all secreted in waves and tides, and a constant wave motion, called peristalsis, pulses through the digestive tract from throat to colon.

The importance of biological rhythms will become more evident, I believe, as clinical data give us a clearer picture of them, but already it is thought that a disruption of the body's natural cycles is a harbinger of disease processes. For example, people who work night shifts and sleep during the day show changes in the daily rhythm of the adrenal hormone cortisol, as well as of certain pituitary hormones. Night workers can adjust their habits to their schedules, but if, as is thought, their cells cannot fully adapt, then the disruptions of biological rhythms may be experienced as a vague sense of disorientation, a susceptibility to colds and infections, and an irritation of the stress response.

It will take medicine a while to determine exactly how the immune system and the hormone system respond to natural cycles, but every observant person sees them all around him. Our emotions change with the seasons, we catch colds in the winter, we feel the spring "in our bones," we become pensive and "riper" in the fall. Our feelings turn to love in spring and return inwards in winter. Various disorders have their own time, too. Ulcers most frequently grow worse and bleed in the months between September and January, for instance. Depression favors the winter too, and its special hours during the day are twilight and just around midnight.

A fascinating discovery in this area has to do with certain people who become chronically depressed, sometimes to the point of feeling suicidal, only in winter. They suffer from what is called the SAD syndrome, or "seasonal affective disorder." The blood of these patients was found to contain high levels of melatonin, a hormone secreted by the pineal gland. In order to lower these levels and relieve the depression, doctors now advise these patients simply to walk in the sunlight more. That is the fascinating part, for the pineal gland's secretions respond to light, even though this gland is securely buried under the skull and surrounded by brain tissue. This gland's behavior seems to be our way of monitoring the year and is apparently due to genetic programming.

Since modern existence is not tied to nature as it once was, our lives can lose touch with inner rhythms. It is possible in a technologized society to set our own clocks. We can work when we want to, sleep when we want to, command practically any food at any time of the year, and stimulate ourselves with television, music, books, and games at any hour. The tempo of this age is part of its evolution, but as a physician, I find that the patients who adapt best to modern speed are those who also respect their body's inner rhythms. This is not news. Really healthy and successful people are frequently those who learned early on to get a full night's sleep, to take time during the day for quiet, to eat at leisure, to rise with the sun and go to bed early.

In fact, because the basic cycle underlying all the others is that of rest and activity, getting sufficient rest is the key to normalizing all our inner rhythms. All therapies for physical and mental disorders include rest. One enemy of rest is continuous stimulation. Inducing a low-level excitation of the brain throughout the day, which many people are unconsciously addicted to, makes it extremely difficult for the waves of rest and activity to function naturally. People suffering from psychological disorders of all types, including those aggravated by fatigue and stress, nearly always display agitation in their thoughts and emotions. They seem to have no rhythms left inside, only excitations. Almost as badly off are people who cannot sleep, who suffer from tension and other signs of stress, heavy users of tobacco, alcohol, or drugs, and those who are victimized by mild chronic depression and worry.

The mental techniques that I discuss in part IV of this book are based upon alternating rest with activity. These techniques bring the profound benefits of perfect health because they put us in touch with the one cycle that upholds all created things. Through your genes, your body has recorded a history of rest and activity that goes back to the creation of the universe. Only by keeping every specific cycle in coordination with every other was the infinite intelligence of nature able to build up levels of evolution from atom to molecule to living tissue to conscious mind.

If you want to move in the direction of creating health, I think it is good to follow the cycles you observe in nature. Wake with your own inner clock, not an alarm. Give yourself some quiet time just after you wake up and just before you go to sleep — in other words, do not instantly flip on the news in the morning or watch TV in bed at night. Work in a quiet area that has a window and exclude music played as a sort of wallpaper in the office. Be fairly quiet and restful after every meal. Take your last food of the day near sundown, or at least three hours before you go to sleep. Lie down for fifteen minutes before dinner and for a few minutes after lunch. Drive quietly without automatically turning on the car radio. Walk in the sunlight every day for at least the few minutes it takes to remind yourself that the universe is our real timekeeper.

28

Having an Open Mind

A FEW YEARS AGO a woman patient was referred to me by a famous endocrinologist, a professor at a well-known medical school in New York and the author of several textbooks on endocrine diseases. The woman turned out to be a close relative of his, and naturally I was surprised to find out her identity. Why wouldn't an authority on endocrine disorders know more than a former student about family ills? I soon discovered the reason. The patient was suffering from a condition known as idiopathic cyclic edema. Such patients, always women, retain an inordinate amount of fluid in their bodies during certain phases of the menstrual cycle, which causes weight gain, bloating, and general discomfort. Although there are a number of theories about it, the cause of the condition is not exactly known.

The only thing a doctor can do, according to standard treatment, is to restrict the patient's salt intake and prescribe diuretics, drugs that increase fluid loss. This may work to some extent, but in general the condition is resistant to treatment. The diuretics also cause leaching of potassium from the body, which can cause muscle weakness and painful cramps.

This patient showed all the characteristics of the disease and had been particularly resistant to all forms of therapy tried so far. She would gain as much as eighteen to twenty pounds and become grotesquely bloated during certain phases of her monthly cycle. Her clothes would not fit her, she felt ugly and depressed, and the diuretics did little more than cause various side effects. The patient was desperate and appeared to be on the verge of a nervous collapse. After I evaluated her, I told her quite honestly that I could do nothing for her except prescribe other kinds of diuretics. She agreed to try them, but the new pills had no effect either, and she continued to suffer from the same symptoms. I wrote a letter to my professor, telling him that I was unable to help.

A few months later, while I was eating in the hospital cafeteria, a very petite, slim, attractive woman came up to greet me — it was my former patient, but totally unrecognizable as her old self. She told me that she had been completely cured of her condition, and she looked it. She told me that she had gone to an acupuncturist. After three or four treatments, all the excess fluid disappeared and never came back again. I was very puzzled. How could a few needles, inserted for a few minutes into different parts of the body which Western medicine says have no real neurological connection, accomplish this?

I took the telephone number of her acupuncturist and gave him a call. He seemed pleased at my interest and spent a long time telling me exactly how the treatment worked. But I came away very disappointed. He spoke of "energy fields" in various parts of the body and how he moved energy from the navel to the liver, and so on. Medically it was gibberish. From my viewpoint, his explanation was totally unscientific and therefore nonsensical. My last thoughts on the case after I hung up were rationalizations — this woman must have been cured by a freak accident or at best by the placebo effect.

Subsequently, however, I came across more patients who had tried traditional Western therapies without obtaining relief, only to gain dramatic results from acupuncture. I could no longer restrain my curiosity and took a closer look at the mechanics of Chinese medicine. I discovered that there was indeed a rational explanation for the effects I had been witnessing. Some of them I could even begin to translate into my own language, the language of modern scientific medicine. Once I started on this tack — in other words, once I opened a new channel for knowledge — I realized that the possibilities for creating health went beyond my training in medical school.

Opening the mind is a real phenomenon. When my mind was closed, obstructed by prejudice, it had not been in touch with the reality of this woman's cure. Therefore the cure had no reality for me, even though I saw it before my eyes. This is the great advantage of having an open mind: it allows reality to show us something new, something hitherto thought impossible, and it does so merely with the power of awareness.

I later got to see the game from the other side. As you will discover in part IV, I became interested in the effects of meditation and learned the simple technique of Transcendental Meditation. Before I started, I had the usual vague prejudices about monks sitting for years in bare Himalayan caves. I discovered from first-hand experience, however, that correct meditation involves a simple mental technique that brings profound benefits to the physiology and completely enlivens the psychophysiological connection. When I try to explain this to other scientists and doctors, they often will not hear of it. Their minds are closed by prejudice; they know "it is all mysticism," and therefore it has no reality for them. Because it is "meditation" and relies on "subjective experience," this technique *must* be unscientific and nonsensical.

We cannot evolve if our minds are closed. This is because we use our minds to evolve. No new knowledge can exist, as we have seen, unless a pathway opens for intelligence to flow through. An open-minded person is simply in the habit of opening new channels. He accepts rather than fears that he will find something new in the world, a discovery that really challenges his prejudices and thus overturns his sacred idols. When intelligence finds a new channel, then more of life flows through us. Bad habits are just the worn-out ruts of the mind, paths that once led to freedom because they opened up new thoughts but that now lead nowhere.

All we have to do is look at the unhealthy minds of prejudiced people to realize that intolerance is toxic. It poisons human growth and makes it impossible for perfect health to flourish. Intelligence is like water — it has to keep running in order to stay pure. An innocent, inquiring, open mind is a prerequisite for healthy living. If you are open to new possibilities in your life, then that alone will give you access to those possibilities — readiness is all.

29

Wonder and Belief

We are inside truth and cannot get outside it.

— Maurice Merleau-Ponty

Why should we not also enjoy an original relation to the universe?

— Ralph Waldo Emerson

THE FACT THAT I am here and now just happens to be an incident in the space-time continuum. A group of atoms took up positions that happened to arrange into further complexities of matter, and the end result was a glob of protoplasm — me. Its constituents have existed since the dawn of the universe and always will exist. Their eternally shifting shapes and forms fill up the manifest cosmos, and there is essentially no difference between them as they reside in me and as they reside in interstellar dust. This world of appearances is not really firm enough to stand on for long. It is what Indian philosophy calls *maya,* "that which is not" or illusion.

The source of illusion is simply change. Our senses do not like change and so have taken on the job of stopping the world. They select a portion of change, lock it "in phase," and thus can perceive it as a fixed reality. But at best these locked-in phases are way stations, and barely that. The universe's vibration never really pauses for an instant. The poet Keats found pleasure in this when he wrote,

The poetry of earth is ceasing never:
. . . .
The poetry of earth is never dead.

As long as we perceive the world as made up of fixed shapes that we believe in, then we are participating in a reality that has ground to a halt. The flow of intelligence has stopped at a way station. When it flows again, reality changes again.

We live in a period when a truly great change is afoot. After centuries of explaining, dissecting, and demystifying nature, science is ready to join the flow once more. In the phrase of the Nobel laureate Ilya Prigogine, science is now mature enough to respect nature. Its next phase, when we may find once more an original relation to the universe, he calls "the re-enchantment of Nature." Enchantment is our natural state. I may be a glob of protoplasm, but in the here and now I cannot cease to wonder at myself and to wonder about wonderment.

To be really healthy is to grow, and you cannot grow unless your viewpoint is innocent, wondering, and, above all, provisional. Nothing is fixed, and the outcome to all of life is open to adventure. There is a marvelous saying in the Talmud, which records that God created the universe with the words, "Let us hope it works!" It is a godlike quality to let life be what it will be. It is a natural capacity in children, who are by nature not bored, cynical, or depressed. When those attitudes creep into our life, you know you are an adult at last.

Modern psychology has attempted to find an age at which the human personality stops growing. So far, no limit has been set. Evolution is an ongoing process that science has found no end to but that it does not yet call intelligent.

At present, the idea of intelligent Nature would be considered an article of faith, a mere belief to a "hard scientist." Science does not hold with belief because it clouds objectivity and therefore is not susceptible to proof. However, the current revolution in science began when certain thinkers started to see that we are not outside nature, and so we cannot divorce nature from what we believe it to be.

Belief and faith are primal forces in nature. We are all believers in something; the values we embrace and the things we hold to be real form our belief system. In the placebo effect, as we saw earlier, the patient's belief in an inert pill brought actual curative results. This is the belief system at work, and only the belief system. Yet the body follows after the belief in order to produce the results. Let us say the patient is told that the pill he is swallowing will absolutely kill pain. If prior to giving him the pill we inject into his system a narcotic antagonist — a drug that blocks the effect of narcotic painkillers — then the placebo effect will not work. This shows that the patient's belief actually produces real molecules of internal painkillers (the endorphins that we have already discussed) which the narcotic antagonist has blocked.

Belief is not limited to pills. The belief can be in anything or anybody and can affect any kind of biological response. In faith healing, for instance, the person must believe that he will be cured, and no doubt so must the healer. In cases of spontaneous remission, the patient must believe in himself. No one, not even the disbelievers, can exist without some belief system. A scientist trained in the traditional objective methodology may say that he has no belief in an infinite intelligence in the universe. Every time he performs an experiment, however, he expresses his belief that there is an order "out there" that can be known and that will give the same results if his experiment is repeated correctly a second time. Without such a belief, no science would be possible.

A higher level of belief is reached when we acknowledge and understand the nature of intelligence on an intellectual level. This is the belief in conscious reasoning. The highest level of belief comes when the mind contacts its own intelligence as an experience. The mind no longer needs reasons to believe in nature's intelligence because it now feels completely inside that intelligence — it is at home with itself. This attainment of belief in its highest manifestation has occasioned man's deep-seated reverence for himself: "Thou shalt decree a thing, and it shall be established unto thee. And light shall shine upon thy ways." Or again, "Ask, and it shall be given you; seek, and ye shall find; knock, and it shall be opened unto you." For the person whose consciousness is such that he truly believes these statements, there can be no failure, no suffering, no ill health, no misery. Such a person can only experience strength, peace, vitality, and wholeness.

What belief can accomplish, then, knows no limits, because the ability of intelligence to create new aspects of reality knows no limits. We are coming closer to what that Vedic sentence meant — the universe is the macrocosm, man is the microcosm. When the gap between our inner life and our outer reality is bridged, nature becomes enchanted once more. A belief in universal intelligence, to quote the teacher and writer Napoleon Hill, "restores health where all else fails, in open defiance of all the rules of modern science. It heals the wounds of sorrow and disappointment regardless of their cause." Belief is an inevitable step toward self-awareness.

30

The Way of Compassion

COMPASSION BEGINS at the source of life. When self-awareness has deepened, when it lightly touches the source of life, compassion appears spontaneously. Awareness has animated it. Compassion is the quality shown by people who can freely express kindness. It is by nature never effortful, never on the surface merely. It is a sympathetic consciousness that takes pity on distress in others and wants to alleviate it. Of all the emotions the human psyche can generate, compassion is the most delicate and the most rewarding.

Like all the tender emotions, if compassion is faithfully described, it is aroused in the hearer. Shakespeare gives these words to Portia in *The Merchant of Venice:*

> The quality of mercy is not strained;
> It droppeth as the gentle rain from heaven
> Upon the place beneath. It is twice blest:
> It blesseth him that gives and him that takes.
> 'Tis mightiest in the mightiest; it becomes

The throned monarch better than his crown.
His scepter shows the force of temporal power,
The attribute to awe and majesty,
Wherein doth sit the dread and fear of kings;
But mercy is above this scept'red sway;
It is enthroned in the hearts of kings,
It is an attribute to God Himself.

Mercy, compassion, and kindness are not accidents of human feeling. They have grown out of universal tendencies in nature according to the process of evolution. All living organisms display behavior patterns that favor the whole over the interests of the individual part. Cells work not for themselves, but for the integrity of the tissue of which they are a part. Tissues likewise work in concert to maintain the integrity of organs, and organs in turn maintain the integrity of the whole organism. Modern biology looks upon this as a sort of genetically programmed altruism. Any part of a living organism is willing to die in order to protect the genetic wholeness of the larger entity.

I am calling this process the beginning of compassion because each cell "sympathetically" senses the need of all other cells and automatically responds to it. As a human trait, compassion may be majestic, but it also shows the healthy continuance of a basic natural instinct. No healing can occur without compassion. It inherently motivates the body and arouses the desire to get well. When this quality is deficient, a doctor comes to provide it. Without compassion, his medical techniques can do very little. The flow of compassion from the physician sets in motion a complex series of biochemical reactions that ultimately effect the cure at the level of physiology.

Norman Cousins puts it exactly when he writes of patients and their "vast collection of emotional needs; they want reassurance; they want to be listened to; they want to feel that it made a difference to the physician, a very big difference, whether they live or die. They want to feel they are in the physician's thoughts." This last, being in a physician's thoughts, I find the most powerful force in doctoring, because it asks a physician for a flow of feeling from the subtlest level. It asks for compassion at the source of life.

Compassion is not what people commonly call altruism. In the end it is even a self-serving mechanism, because it restores and renews the person who gives it. It heals the healer. To have a deficiency of compassion means to be isolated from the emotions of others, and that is a dangerous, disease-provoking state. Even though compassion is inherent, it wants to grow and evolve; therefore, it can be cultivated. Here, the Tibetan Buddhist lama Tarthang Tulku Rinpoche speaks of cultivating compassion:

> Everything is extraordinarily inter-related. As one realizes this, each relationship becomes based on feelings of love — not calculated love, but a natural friendliness to all beings, a natural openness based on a natural understanding of inter-relationship. Gradually the whole idea of self-motivation disappears, and one sees that when you have no self-motivation or self-interest, then all your problems get solved. There no longer exists any individual problem.

I find this inspiring because it shows how the ideal state of mind — "I have no problems" — grows in one simply as a part of life. It is not forced or striven for. What is necessary, as Tarthang goes on to say, is to see other people as a part of your own life:

> The more I learn of other problems, the more my own problems automatically dissolve. So it is important to observe other people's problems. . . . Knowledge of the other person increases self-knowledge; self-knowledge increases compassion; compassion increases knowledge of the other person. It is a very tight circle, which can only be entered through giving up excessive pre-occupation with one's own problems.

The various schools of modern depth psychology, beginning with psychoanalysis, have been guilty to some extent of fostering this excessive preoccupation with our own problems. The East may not have attained its ideals of enlightenment throughout society, but it has benefited from having the concept, as part of the larger idea of enlightenment, that one is dedicated to all sentient beings; Buddha himself is everywhere known as "the compassionate one." Keeping track of one's own problems is not a sign of self-development. It bespeaks a narrow, stunted vision, and compassion is the way out.

Through the eyes of compassion, all of us are equalized. We are parts of the infinite life of the universe and deserve an equal place in it. This reality has been seen clearly whenever the doors of perception have been cleansed. I cannot say as well what I mean as this poem does from the great Bengali poet, Rabindranath Tagore:

> Upagupta, the disciple of Buddha, lay asleep in
>   the dust by the city wall of Mathura.
> Lamps were all out, doors were all shut, and
>   stars were all hidden by the murky sky of August.
> Whose feet were those tinkling with anklets,
>   touching his breast of a sudden?
> He woke up startled, and the light from a woman's
>   lamp fell on his forgiving eyes.
> It was the dancing girl, starred with jewels,
> Wearing a pale blue mantle, drunk with the wine
>   of her youth.
> She lowered her lamp and saw the young face
>   austerely beautiful.
> "Forgive me, young ascetic," said the woman,
> "Graciously come to my house. The dusty earth
>   is not a fit bed for you."
> The young ascetic answered, "Woman,
>   go on your own way;
> When the time is ripe I will come to you."
> Suddenly the black night showed its teeth
>   in a flash of lightning.
> The storm growled from the corner of the sky, and
> The woman trembled in fear of some unknown danger.

A year had not yet passed.
It was the evening of a day in April, in spring season.
The branches of the wayside trees were full of
 blossom.
Gay notes of a flute came floating in the
 warm spring air from afar.
The citizens had gone to the woods for the
 festival of flowers.
From the mid sky gazed the full moon on the
 shadows of the silent town.
The young ascetic was walking along the lonely street,
While overhead the love-sick koels uttered from the
 mango branches their sleepless plaint.
Upagupta passed through the city gates, and
 stood at the base of the rampart.
Was that a woman lying at his feet in the
 shadow of the mango grove?
Struck with black pestilence, her body
 spotted with sores of small-pox,
She had been hurriedly removed from the town
To avoid her poisonous contagion.
The ascetic sat by her side, took her head
 on his knees,
And moistened her lips with water, and
  smeared her body with sandal balm.
"Who are you, merciful one?" asked the woman.
"The time, at last, has come to visit you, and
 I am here," replied the young ascetic.

31

A Vision of Wholeness and Love

Love is not a mere impulse; it must contain truth, which
is law.

— Rabindranath Tagore

THE MECHANICS of evolution are the mechanics of love. We were
all conceived as a thought of love and desire that became bound
into minute genetic matter. When we were newborns, the same
love nurtured us, and our first conscious thoughts of ourselves
were so entwined with our mother's love that there was no awareness of separation. If the force of love can conceive life, nurture it,
and give it identity, then it must be part of the intelligence that *is*
us.

The self-aware mind is simply one that continues to use its intelligence with love. It can at times even have an experience of
pure love. No matter in what age or place, the records of all such
experiences have an undeniable similarity. The description is always of a primal moving force, at once dynamic and all-pervasive,
that cannot be separated from "wholeness." Those few who have
sustained the experience of pure love are the guides of humanity.

Yet the same guide is embodied in our cells, and we literally can
have no conscious life or impulse of intelligence without consulting it. Love guides intelligence. It is like a common thread that we
cannot drop from our hands so long as we are in the stream of

evolution. The thread leads from our selves across the threshold of our thoughts onto the portico of the universe. Everyone carries his piece of the thread in a strand of DNA that marks him as an irreplaceable part of existence. In delicate moments of refined attention, one can feel love as the gentle tug of evolution. It makes the process of living go forward simply because it *wants* to go forward. Evolution in this sense is not a "relentless force" but a sequence of innocent desires.

Love is so innocent and direct. It delights in what it looks at, and at its purest, it recognizes no higher purpose than delight. That is why innocent awareness of other people has an actual power and exerts such a transforming influence — it is love. Simply to see that love infuses all of nature, which is the realization contained in every peak experience, makes life creative. One touch of love, and the raw material of life is shaped to a purpose. Love is a creative force, and through creation one seeks joy and immortality.

Love's strongest conviction is of unity. The mind can be overwhelmed to see this in a flash, but it is also there in the everyday state of things. Everyone loves his house, his child, his garden, yet taken to its conclusion, the same feeling becomes infinite: "I love this universe, it is mine." The idea is expressed innocently and beautifully by Swami Satchidananda:

> One day I was working in the field, and I hurt my finger. I could have ignored it, but I cleaned it and bandaged it. If I had ignored it and the finger got infected, my entire body would have suffered. The same way, if we feel that we are parts of the cosmic body, the entire universe, how can we stop from loving the other parts?

From this simple reasoning springs the necessity to set life on a higher plane. If differences are an illusion produced in the head, then seeing the reality of nondifference restores reality. Love restores reality. The swami goes on:

> Once you feel that you are a part of the whole, that you belong to the whole, and the whole world belongs to you, that very feeling makes you love, and that very love brings forth healing. . . . No healer can

heal without that universal love. If you realize that you are not just an individual, but a part of the whole universe, you will not be afraid of anyone. A fearless man lives always, a fearful man dies every day, every minute.

Does thinking that I am part of the whole universe make a difference? As a mere thought, I do not believe so. But a "realization" is more than a thought. It signifies that a moment of awareness has changed reality. Something new wakes up when awareness touches it.

One of the most audacious thinkers in the vanguard of the "new physics," David Bohm, has proposed the awareness of unity as a scientific hypothesis. He has coined the phrase *implicate order* and used it to connect all physical events in the universe to one another, so that a detailed study of any one part would in principle give total knowledge of every other part. This implies that people contact a universal reality when they love or are visited by "mystical" insights. They actually are joining others at the level of a unified consciousness. Bohm describes it this way:

> Even if a hundred people were able to perceive the deepest stratum of reality and tap into the collective mind — the ego would vanish for these people, and they would form a single consciousness, just as the parts of a highly integrated person are integrated as one.

The new physics has also offered the idea that our universe — the cosmic body — was whole to begin with and always will be. It may be that science will conclude that the boiling currents of matter and energy have no reality at all, or a poor, secondhand reality, compared to the underlying orderliness that keeps wholeness whole. So far as human wisdom has ever been able to express it, the true reality of "wholeness" is love. Finding the same implicate order in nature and inside ourselves is not a chance discovery. Science is verifying through its belief system the same idea that a sensitive person can find in his own awareness — "We are inside truth and cannot get outside it," as Merleau-Ponty put it. A man who can actually believe in "my universe" will see it as a universe of pure intelligence guided by love.

These are all wonderful and inspiring sentiments; we find them in the words of every saint in every religion. We may agree with them, we may take them seriously and even literally, but who is capable of turning them to practical use?

Love is meant to be cultivated. Love has been grasped in every awareness but not completely used. The use of love is to heal. When it flows without effort from the depth of the self, love creates health. Children deprived of warm mothering at infancy can only be healed through love and compassion. Their bodies are able to reverse years of stressful functioning and emotional starvation if only the contact with love is renewed. In that sense, love is quite practical. It comes into use the instant we feel it in our awareness.

Loving, compassionate people — those whose intelligence is used with love — are in general the healthiest and happiest people. They will always tell you that their love is ultimately selfish, because it restores and renews them every day. When life is full, it is only love, and when awareness is full, it brings only love. Every impulse of intelligence in our awareness starts its journey from the source of life as love and nothing else.

We can set our lives on a higher plane of awareness, and then we will understand the simplicity that is love. It will not be a thought, hope, sentiment, or dream. It will be part of us, the breath of our life. As we will discover in the last part of this book, bringing our awareness to its source is easy, because that is where awareness naturally wants to be.

IV

Toward a Higher Reality: Meditation and Metamorphosis

32

Reality, Manifest and Unmanifest

Reality is a symbol.
— Fazal Inayat-Khan

WE TEND TO REGARD THINGS that we can perceive with our senses as real. Things that are not readily available to our senses we generally think of as unreal or imaginary. Not only that, we are apt to grade the degree of "realness" in an object in proportion to the number of senses it can stimulate. A warm, fragrant, solid, moving thing seems quite vivid and therefore more real than, for instance, a microbe. At bottom, we have a bias for solidity. If something is supposed to be real, then let me touch it.

Because our notions of reality are constructed at a subjective level, it is quite easy to see why we stick with the idea that some things are real and some are not. The most real things to us, after all, are ourselves. After a course in philosophy, we may doubt the existence of everything else in the cosmos, but we are pretty sure of our own existence. The more an object does to remind us of ourselves, the more ready we are to admit that it too is real and has a valid existence. Higher education changes this casual yardstick only a little. Scientists for the most part do not accept the existence of anything that is not readily manifest to the senses.

Of course, science has gone a tremendously long way to bring more things into the range of the senses. With the help of a radio receiver, we can extend our sense of hearing very far. Eavesdropping on the twitter of outer space is now a possibility. Without the aid of radio, we would have no idea that such sounds are coming to earth all the time, and we would feel justified in saying that they do not exist. The telescopes that enormously increase the range of what we can see now peer at stars whose light started out toward us millions of years ago. Therefore, by extending sight the telescope also crosses the time barrier to extend time. If we are seeing light from a star that has subsequently burned out, we could claim that the telescope is seeing something that is not even in existence.

It becomes immediately obvious that we are constructing reality according to our perception. Rabindranath Tagore, who was not merely a poet but a speculative thinker too, wrote that "it is almost a truism to say that the world is what we perceive it to be. We imagine that our mind is a mirror, that it is more or less accurately reflecting what is happening outside us. On the contrary our mind itself is the principal element of creation. The world, while I am perceiving it, is being incessantly created for myself in time and space." The perceptions we use to judge reality come from the senses, but all that they pick up — the fragrance of a rose, the sight of the full moon, the touch of fog — is relayed to the mind. However much we extend our perceptions with quasar detectors or electron microscopes, all perception ultimately occurs in the mind. If you stand on your head at the beach, you will see something quite real to your eyes when you witness the ocean flowing over the sky, but your mind is not fooled. It is your mind that ultimately sees, hears, tastes, smells, and touches.

Reality in its final sense is constructed in the mind — the mind makes reality. Outside our perceptions, thoughts, and experiences, reality has no validity. The shape, size, appearance, or any other attribute of an object is purely a subjective quality. We create our reality.

Let us take an example. Imagine for a moment that the human eye is equipped with a square lens instead of the oval one it actually has. Just this one change in our ordinary sensory apparatus would completely alter the appearance of the whole world. A marble perceived through the square lens of the eye might now have the shape of a pencil, and rolling the marble with our fingers would be very different from rolling a smooth, regular sphere, which is what we are completely used to and take for granted. As long as all human beings possessed this square-shaped lens, we would all accept the new shape of marbles, and we would think that the sight of pencil-shaped objects rolling around and feeling smooth to the touch was absolutely normal.

Another species, a rabbit, for instance, would perceive the marble according to its own eye structure, and for it, that would be reality. The chameleon turns each of its eyes on a separate swivel rather than together, so we cannot remotely imagine its world; its vision has nothing in common with the way sight is set up in our nervous system. A shark can apparently smell blood from a fish killed several miles away, which we cannot imagine either, since our noses do not even work under water.

Going back to the marble, suppose that we ask what the "real" shape of the marble is. The answer is that there is no "real" shape. The marble has no shape independent of the perceiver. It is the perception that gives the marble its shape. The same holds for all the other senses. It takes only a little jump to conclude that the marble has no perceptible existence independent of the perceiver. It would not exist as it does without a mind to perceive it.

Perception is not only shaped by the senses and interpreted by the mind. It depends on past experiences as they are stored in the physiology. A simple experiment conducted with kittens by Helmut and Spinelli demonstrates what I mean. Three batches of kittens were raised in three separate environments. One set was put in a room whose walls were painted with horizontal stripes, and that was all that the kittens were permitted to see. A second batch of kittens grew up in an environment of vertical stripes, and the third in one that was entirely white, with no markings of any kind.

When these kittens became adult cats, each batch perceived a world different from the world perceived by the others. Those exposed only to horizontal stripes as kittens could see horizontal shapes perfectly well, but they could not see anything that was vertical. They bumped into furniture legs, for example, as though they were not there — because for these cats they were not. The batch of cats living in a vertical world had exactly the opposite problem, while the cats from the completely white world failed to develop adequate adult vision at all and therefore had the worst disorientation visually. This was not a question of what the cats believed in. Their brains could only perceive a limited and selective part of the visual continuum that nature offers. This is true for all of us.

Other experiments have led to similar results. When newborn monkeys had one eye patched and the other left open for a period of time, the brain connections to the blind eye dwindled and finally failed altogether, while the ones to the open eye flourished. Also, it was found that the timing of perceptual development is crucial. Kittens are born blind, and if their eyes are bandaged just for the short period, a few days long, when eyesight begins, they will be blind for life. All of these experiments show that the electrical patterns stored in the nervous system from previous experience serve to build up the connections and receptors physically responsible for perception. So the very structure of the brain itself, the seat of perception, depends upon our past experience of the world. We begin to see the truth in the words of the ancient mystic Rumi, "New organs of perception come into being as the result of necessity."

However, we seem now to have the snake biting its own tail. We say that experience shapes perception, but we started off by saying that perception shapes experience. It is a very tight circle. What we need to realize is that perception and experience are both *created* by the mind. The eye and what it sees, the ear and what it hears, the tongue and what it tastes, the nose and what it smells, the nerves and what they feel, all are made in the mind. The material world does not exist independently of the mind.

To put it broadly, without the mind there is no material universe. It is quite literally a mirage, an ephemeral thing that the mind has created. Though not tangible or even manifest to the senses, it is the mind that is displaying itself through the material world and its infinite number of manifested objects. The objects possess at best a secondhand reality that is no reality at all compared to what is real — unmanifest mind. The mind is the creative source of the world; you and I are the source of the world. Our entire reality springs from us, our ideas, our notions of the real. Reality is a symbolic manifest expression of an unmanifest idea.

To create something "out there," all we have to do is first agree between ourselves that a certain reality exists out there, and then that agreement between us would construct that reality. In the last chapter we mentioned David Bohm's hypothesis that human beings all share one consciousness at some deep level. This collective consciousness is what you and I are putting to work when we agree to construct reality together. Our collective consciousness at a deep level, well below the level of the opinions that we can superficially change, agrees that this reality exists. It has sunk its roots into our physiology, and we have built a world up around it.

Before anything can become a reality, then, it must exist in seed form as a flicker, a perturbation in collective consciousness. This perturbation happens well out of sight and first manifests itself as the faintest notion we can have in our minds: "I am." This is just our tendency to think that we are real, the idea this chapter started off with. As soon as "I am" is accepted, then millions upon millions of things can show up on the scene. They manifest themselves as faint emotions, faint ideas, then stronger ideas and groups of beliefs, and finally as a full-blown world.

Reality is the final result, for better or worse. If the collective consciousness — that is, you and I — agrees upon the existence of wars, then we have wars. Wars are the manifestations of a kind of perturbation in the collective consciousness called stress. If we did not agree to have wars, wars would not exist. Right now, everything that you and I and everyone else agrees is horrible, at some other level, in the depths of collective consciousness, took its reality because we agreed to it. We get sick, we grow old, we become disabled because of our notions and ideas that these are the realities of life. We were told that, we accept that, so we go on creating that. If we did not accept those notions first, we would not necessarily accept sickness, age, and infirmity as reality.

To give just a passing example, we all accept that if one runs, one gets tired. It is a physiological fact. Yet certain Indians of the Sierra Madre in Mexico run long distances, sometimes more than fifty miles, as a normal part of their culture. Everyone likes to do it, though for us it is hard to imagine running a distance twice as long as a marathon. The Indians even kick a ball as they go. An American physiologist recorded the heart rate of the winner immediately after one of these races. The instruments recorded that his heart was beating more slowly than it was when he started.

The key to the reality of our universe lies in the fact that we are choosing it. Before we choose, we need to realize the mechanics whereby our ideas manifest themselves as reality. Once we become fully aware of those mechanics, then we can promote into reality only those ideas that are evolutionary. We could choose courage, hope, love, peace, health — even immortality is not out of the question — and they would become our realities. Up to now, however, we have firmly chosen fear, hatred, greed, envy, war, sickness, and death. Without our giving the matter any conscious thought, these have been imposed on us by the collective consciousness. Our bodies and what they can do, our brains and what they can conceive, are living expressions of received opinions. If we are to change them for the better, then we must first learn how to change collective consciousness. As history abundantly makes clear, you cannot change reality with good intentions alone.

We are pure consciousness at the source, before any perturbations or any flicker of ideas arise. By diving deep into our source, we will discover the mechanics of creation. Once that is found, then we can choose. We will really be free to think, and so we can think peace, perfect health, youthfulness — any reality we choose will be under our control. Having good ideas in our own minds is obviously a necessary step, but they will not become full-fledged realities until they replace the wrong ideas entrenched in collective consciousness. Indeed, collective consciousness will not seem real to the skeptical mind until we show that we can actually *do* something with it. Only the things that appear to the senses tend to be accepted as reality. Therefore, we must look next to the force that is capable of shaping all reality, which is intelligence.

33

The Nature and Range of Intelligence

> The range of creative intelligence is:
>   From smaller than the smallest to larger than
>   the largest,
>   From unmanifest through all manifestations to
>   unmanifest — unbounded, infinite, eternal,
>   From Here to Here,
>   From "I" to "I,"
>   From seed to seed,
>   From fullness to fullness.
>
> — Maharishi Mahesh Yogi

BEFORE WE MAKE INTELLIGENCE INFINITE, let us see how big it already is. The word has many different applications. Depending on your viewpoint, *intelligence* can mean the ability to learn or understand, or to deal with new or trying situations; the ability to apply knowledge to manipulate one's environment; or to think abstractly, to organize information coherently, and to use that information to solve a problem. All of these are valid meanings of intelligence. But intelligence also has the ring of being a human quality. Because we think of ourselves as intelligent, we tend to limit the idea of intelligence to a specific human ability, the power of reason.

But intelligence is much more than the ability to reason with the intellect. Certainly the ability to reason is the conscious capacity that sets mankind above other creatures in nature and serves to measure "higher" intelligence in terms of intellectual prowess. But everything in nature, starting with a single particle or a bundle of energy, contains information. From this information it derives some know-how. At the very least, it knows how to be a particle and how to interact properly with other inanimate parts of the universe. Any know-how that can be used is a sign of intelligence. Itzhak Bentov, writing about the basic nature of the cosmos, defined consciousness as "the ability of a system to respond to a stimulus." I consider that also a workable definition of intelligence at its simplest level, where intelligence and consciousness cannot be separated.

Following this definition, the level of intelligence that a system exhibits would then depend on the *range* of responses it could show when it was stimulated. The more complex, varied, and innovative a system shows itself to be, the more intelligent we could consider it. This measure of intelligence is mechanical, but it has one great advantage: all intelligence would be measured by the same standard. We would avoid thinking that any single sort of intelligence (that of humans, of course) is better than that of another because it is simply different. But we still might fall into the error of placing a "simple" thing like an electron at the bottom of the totem pole because it is less intelligent than, for instance, a whale. We need to remember that without the electron the whale has no existence and therefore no intelligence to be proud of.

An electron seems capable of only a limited range of responses. Basically, it chooses an orbit around the atom's nucleus and stays there unless stimulated to jump to a higher orbit. When the stimulus is removed, the electron automatically falls back into place. Even this simple response, however, causes the emission of one photon of light, so we see immediately that any condition in the universe in which there is light requires the organized behavior of electrons acting in incredibly diverse situations.

So it is not fair of us to isolate the electron at all. It is a complex system within the complex system of the atom, which in turn behaves inside the complex system of molecules. We can mount up the totem pole until we reach the human brain, and there we find a system capable of infinite responses. Its limitless intelligence, however, is fully coordinated with the electron at the bottom. Electrons are "intelligent" enough not to misbehave. If they did, the totem pole would fall over — there would be chaos.

Yet the human mind is creative in its intelligence, while the electron is apparently mechanical. Creative thought is nothing but a new or previously undocumented response to a variety of stimuli. Even an original idea is mechanical, in that it depends upon the correct operation of brain tissue, enzymes, hormones, electrical connections, and so on, cascading down the chain of intelligence to the bottom. Some responses look very different from others — walking down the road does not look like enzymes locking onto receptors on the cell wall — but there is a common linkage that organizes and gives purpose to every response from the smallest to the greatest, and that is intelligence.

Creative intelligence at the human level is the final expression of know-how gathered over time throughout nature. As we have already seen, the information in our DNA is like an encyclopedia of all the evolution in the universe. The simple information of the electron had to be preserved and passed on to the atom, which built on it and passed along its information to the molecule, and so on throughout time. All this infinite, universal intelligence serves evolution. So far as science can tell, there are no spare parts in the universe. Anything that could exist has been used. The stream of evolution swept everything along and organized it into the way it *has to be* in order for us to live and think our creative thoughts.

The human brain is the glory of nature, not simply because it is complex and we all happen to have one, but because it can evolve without end. That means that all the intelligence in the universe is capable of responding to the growth of the human mind. Charles Darwin, the father of modern theories of evolution, wrote, "In many cases, the continued development of a part, for instance, the beak of a bird, or the teeth of a mammal, would not aid the species in gaining its food, or for any other object, but with man we can see no definite limit to the continued development of the brain and mental faculties, as far as advantage is concerned."

Man focuses the infinite intelligence of the universe. If we do not usually think so, it may be because we think that intellect created intelligence. It is the other way around: intelligence created intellect. Naturally, because it is only one manifestation of intelligence, the intellect is limited; after several centuries of study, we do not even know, for instance, how our own organs work. Intelligence, however, is not limited. It is all-pervasive and infinite. It expresses the infinite organizing power in nature. On a small scale it shows itself as the electron's willingness to behave; on the larger scale, it shows itself as the great accomplishments of human creativity. Each level of intelligence is different, yet all act in infinite correlation with each other: "When an electron vibrates, the universe shakes."

Modern science investigates all the parts of nature's endless order, but it has not looked until recently into the wholeness of nature (we will see what it has recently discovered about the mechanics of creation in the next chapter). In the East there is a great tradition of knowledge about wholeness but not in the form we call science. In India, for instance, the great sages have spoken of intelligence by consulting their own awareness. Here is a passage from the Bhagavad Gita that explains the rungs of intelligence as nature has arranged them in man: "The senses, they say, are subtle; more subtle than the senses is mind; yet finer than mind is intellect; that which is beyond even the intellect is 'He.' " By "He," the sage means the source of intelligence before a thought even flickers, in other words, the self.

The great Eastern traditions still have modern figures to speak for them. Maharishi Mahesh Yogi, who has taught about infinite human potential for three decades, particularly emphasizes the "science" of creative intelligence. His language is not metaphorical or archaic, but quite literal: "The galaxies do not just run about here and there at random; there is an order in creation; there is system in creation. Without the fundamental value of intelligence all this order and growth would not be found." I became interested in his approach to intelligence because, first, he takes it as self-evident that order is everywhere around us and can be viewed as a whole. Second, he believes that when a person arrives at the source of his own intelligence, he can change reality in the direction of health, happiness, knowledge, and peace; Maharishi calls this "the increasing steps of progress towards the fullness of life."

What we want to find out are the mechanics that enable us to create reality. The mechanics begin in our mind as a faint awareness of "I am," and then by progressive steps the fullness of our world emerges. Although it seems astonishing to think that we can learn to change reality from the level of awareness, in fact we are creating it at every moment. The mechanics of creative intelligence are not just "out there" making galaxies, photons, redwood trees, and howler monkeys. The flow of creative intelligence moves through us, enabling us to be "in phase" with our own version of reality.

Maharishi Mahesh Yogi is not merely a philosopher discussing creative intelligence. As we will see in chapter 35, he proposes very specific techniques for effortlessly bringing our awareness back to the source of thought. Once established there, we can learn to control the flow of intelligence that is ours, and in that way all the desirable qualities of human existence — love, compassion, health, personal fulfillment — will increase in our lives. I should mention also that what we are looking into is not just Eastern in origin. Henri Bergson, a French philosopher, won a Nobel Prize in 1927 for writings that expounded his theories of "creative evolution," only to fall out of notice for the simple reason that experimental science could not validate that what he claimed had any practical basis. What was lacking was a technique that made creative intelligence a living reality, something that the Eastern traditions have spent centuries perfecting.

It is possible to have a science of creative intelligence because intelligence works systematically throughout nature. Its range may be "from smaller than the smallest to larger than the largest," to use the classic Indian description, but certain principles hold true at every level. To name just a few of them, intelligence expresses orderliness; it unites parts into a unified wholeness; it alternates in rhythms of rest and activity; it progresses effortlessly by removing all obstacles in its path; it is entirely contained in the smallest parts of a system; and it displays infinite stability alongside infinite adaptability.

As an endocrinologist, I am fascinated with the way that the human body perfectly exhibits these principles. Just to take orderliness, for example, I can quote Claude Bernard, generally acknowledged as the father of modern physiology; he speaks of the rigid laws of physics and biochemistry that the processes of the body must adhere to, but then he observes that "they subordinate themselves and succeed one another in a pattern, and according to a law which pre-exists; they repeat themselves with order, regularity, constancy, and they harmonize in such a manner as to bring about the organization and growth of the individual." This perfect expression of order and growth Bernard found in all animals and plants — it is a principle of intelligence found throughout nature.

Taking the endocrine system to illustrate the other principles, it is easy to see that this system alternates in cycles of rest and activity; biology is constantly exploring new and elegant "periodicities" that regulate the secretion of all our hormones. The endocrine system contains various parts, the different glands, separated over considerable distances in the body, but they act as one network, a whole connected by the sequential triggering of hormonal pathways, each one exquisitely sensitive to the needs of the entire physiology. The hormones themselves are secreted and regulated without effort by the autonomic nervous system, and in only fractions of a second they can reverse their processes to deal with any change in the internal environment. In that way we can say that they are infinitely stable in their precise functioning, yet infinitely flexible in the situations that the body can call on them for — every single thought or action calls up a unique response from the endocrine network.

The endocrine system would appear to be a specific solution that nature has evolved for the specific conditions of the human body. But in fact, cellular biology is discovering that the processes in our hormone system are repeated in similar patterns throughout the web of life. The mechanism for using glucose, for instance, is the same in a bacterium as in a human cell. And insulin, which plays a key role in our metabolic processes, appears in the evolutionary chain across eons of time, from cold-blooded fish to man.

Not just our brain, but every cell in our body displays this same complexity of intelligence. Every cell perceives a world around it; every one of them "remembers" the past and "predicts" the future in its biochemical responses; and thanks to DNA, every cell contains all the information that makes up the intelligence that is you. To speak of a flow of infinite intelligence in us is to speak quite literally, for it governs every cell and tissue. It is in our fingernails, our teeth, our intestines, and our glands. It sets our biological clock as precisely as the one in a migrating monarch butterfly or in a white dwarf star. The rivers flowing to the ocean, the bees attracted to nectar, and the eagle soaring on an August thermal share the same principles of creative intelligence with us. Life is not our prerogative.

But it *is* our unique ability to become aware of these principles and to use them according to our desires. All intelligence is interconnected and the same, only expressing itself in different forms. To control intelligence in our awareness is to control all intelligence. The project of perfecting human creativity to that extent is more important for our well-being than any other project we can conceive. We have begun this project by examining the nature of intelligence. Now we will look at the mechanics of creation. They are the control switches in nature that give us the power to alter reality.

34

The Mechanics of Creation

Curving back within myself I create again and again.
— Bhagavad Gita

CREATION IS A FUNCTION of intelligence. Some process of change is implied, generally a change that causes something new to appear. By the mechanics of creation, I simply mean the process of change. If we can grasp how intelligence actually goes through the process of change, then we can use intelligence to cause change. We know that we want to create a reality for ourselves that is beneficial; therefore, we do not have to restrict ourselves to creation at a mechanical level, for instance at the level where electrons interact. Instead, we will take the perspective of ourselves, the level where our intelligence already creates change in all aspects of living. And in particular, since we want to create health, happiness, and self-fulfillment, we will want to know how the mind-body connection can function to give us these results.

Human intelligence does not create on one level only. Consider the Empire State Building; its creation involved the architect's designs, the consultation of all sorts of engineers and builders, the physical work of construction, and so on. But at the subtlest level, it was collective consciousness that brought the Empire State Building into existence — the orderly, coherent desires of separate individuals were coordinated and directed to one purpose. Or to put it even more simply, a thought was shared and brought into physical existence.

In order for the building to become real, someone had to move from the realm of thought to the realm of action. Cement and steel had to be moved. But intelligence can work much more directly. Let us say that a patient is diagnosed with a malignancy and is eventually cured. As this book has shown you, the way to that cure can be either indirect or direct. If the doctor prescribes treatment by radiation and drugs, then he is creating a cure from the outside. Of course it is really the body that is creating a healthy state for itself, but the outside intelligence of the doctor brings in curative agents to help the body to act. Malignancies can be healed, however, by intelligence acting directly. The woman described earlier in this book who treated herself by using the Simonton visualization techniques was cured by applying a conscious mental routine that opened a channel for health. Another patient, Mrs. Di Angelo, used her intelligence even more directly. She effected her cure merely by having a desire, "I never want to be sick again, and so I never will be sick again."

Which level of creating the cure was most desirable? Obviously, the last one was. The most efficient mechanics of creation are those in which intelligence acts within itself. If we can alter reality from that deep, subtle level, then the grosser levels will all follow along automatically. A desire in the mind, acting directly through the mind-body connection, can effortlessly translate itself into a physical reality in the body. In this case it was a cure of a malignant disease process, but it could be any change in the direction of health and self-fulfillment.

Already we have discovered the most profound laws of creation that intelligence works through. The first law is that intelligence works by itself to change itself; nothing outside the system needs to be brought in because nothing is outside the domain of intelligence to begin with — intelligence is all-pervasive. This principle is called self-referral. The next law says that intelligence can find a way to accomplish anything. It does not matter at all if medicine tells us that a cure is impossible. For every thought we might have, nature can provide a direct way to accomplish its fulfillment. We can call this the existence of all possibilities.

Third, the intelligence that accomplished the cure worked in an orderly, automatic, and integrated fashion. No matter which cure you look at, the body's systems went about the process of healing by doing one thing after another in just the right sequence and without the need for the conscious mind to intervene.

In other words, once a thought sets up the initial condition, all the mechanics of carrying out the thought work by themselves. Maharishi Mahesh Yogi puts great emphasis on this principle; he calls it the principle of "the highest first." It is really the principle of efficiency, because it says that the best way to get to a goal is the quickest, shortest, and easiest way. If we resort to medicinal drugs, then nature accepts that as a condition and works through the specific mechanisms of the drug therapy. But these are very weak, slow, laborious, complex, and sometimes painful in their action. If you could activate a cure simply with a thought, as in the placebo effect, then nature takes that just as seriously as an initial condition, but it can work out a cure much more quickly, more smoothly, and with less pain and complication than drugs call for.

Finding a way to have nature do all the work is the greatest secret in the mechanics of creation. Finding this way involves believing in all the other principles of creation, because without a belief that intelligence is infinite, orderly, and capable of all possibilities, you will inevitably decide that only one way to a goal is right, the one your view of reality has ingrained in you. You will always use drugs or radiation, for instance, because you refuse to believe that nature works cures in any other way. Of course this is the same as saying that no one before the twentieth century ever recovered from cancer, which is absurd. So the principle of the highest first makes a tremendous difference in all situations where you have a choice of which path your creativity will take.

What we have learned about the mechanics of creation goes even further than this. Because nature operates through intelligence, it is bringing knowledge to solve a problem, and in setting up the mechanics of solving the problem, nature has to correlate all sorts of different parts. In the case of a cure, the mind-body connection works through the immune system, the hormone system, the cardiovascular system, and so on. But the degree of knowledge being used and the amount of correlation that the mind-body connection is capable of are not the same from case to case. Drugs, for example, interfere with the body — that is why they have side effects — and force it to cooperate with the chemical properties of the drug. So the direct nondrug cures are more effective because they exhibit more complete, holistic knowledge and more pervasive correlation.

The principle of creation that this conclusion brings out is that nature contains infinite organizing power and infinite correlation. In the operation of the universe, nothing short of infinite knowledge and infinite correlation is being used all the time; there are no spare parts in the universe. But through our conscious choice we can limit nature to very narrow channels. Before opening the channel of electricity, we could only create light with fire. The most effective creative mind is the one that allows maximum knowledge and maximum correlation to spring forth from nature's unlimited supply. This becomes very important when we consider what are called "higher states" of consciousness, because the amount of knowledge and organizing power your mind can use depends directly on your awareness of how much there is. You have to be aware that electricity exists before you can use it; you have to be aware of your infinite creative potential before you can use that as well. In fact, only awareness can activate it for you.

None of these principles will seem valid until you accept their reality. For modern people, the only measure of validity is science; it has taken the place of faith, authority, and instinct. What are the mechanics of creation so far as science is concerned? The creation of material objects, whether on the scale of the universe or on that of the photon, is the domain of physics. What it has to say about creation will be very supportive of the views I am putting forth about mind and body. In particular, we want to look at the "new physics," the era that began with the work of Einstein and his great European colleagues.

The new physics totally altered the idea of the solid, predictable reality that people took for granted in the West since the time of Aristotle. In the old view, time and space were separate entities, and objects moved through them like balls on a billiard table, in other words, following fixed paths that the senses could detect. Now we speak of "space-time" as one continuous thing, and we routinely take for granted, ever since the dawn of atomic power, that matter can be changed to energy, causing it to disappear from the billiard table and go off into nowhere. The famous uncertainty principle formulated by Werner Heisenberg tells us that we cannot even know the "real" properties of an object with any certainty, because the process of observation actually changes the nature of the object being observed.

The working out of the new physics has taken most of this century to accomplish and has required the intelligence of eminently brilliant minds. The new world view that their thought produced has reached popular acceptance only in the past fifteen years; without some knowledge of mathematics, the implications of this new world view are quite difficult to grasp. Much is still in dispute, and physicists spend their lives in theoretical controversy. However, it is possible to extrapolate certain basic ideas and apply them to ourselves, not as rigorous scientists, but as interested lay people who want to deal with reality as it really is.

I will give in simple form some of the initial findings of modern physics. One is that objects have no distinct solidity at any level. The particles that make up objects are actually transformations of energy; as such, they are basically waves, but they can behave like particles, in other words like matter, under certain conditions. The famous example given by Bertrand Russell had to do with his writing table. He pointed out that the table was not solid at all. It was made up of energy and empty space, with space occupying more than 99.9999 percent of the total. What made it seem solid is the fact that our senses make it that way. We have already discussed the importance of this.

Secondly, no particle or bundle of energy is isolated. They are all tiny outcroppings of wave functions that extend infinitely in time and space. Like tips of the iceberg, they crop up from a vaster reality that is out of sight. In the case of matter and energy, most of the wave literally exists out of time and space altogether. All the objects of the universe have sprung out of the unmanifest void and will one day go back into it. The void itself is the "real" reality, and anything we can imagine existing is already there in what physicists call "virtual" form. In fact, it is possible to calculate that everything that could exist in the place where you now sit actually does exist, but in virtual form. Millions of realities inhabit your room, only your senses exclude them in favor of the scene you accept as real here and now. So far as the new physics is concerned, even the past and future are enfolded in your room already.

Your chair, your walls, and your body are mere probabilities that have cropped up from the eternal, infinite, and unmanifest field that underlies the universe and keeps it organized. When you drop a tennis ball, it falls to the floor, but there is a small, completely precise probability that it would go straight up to the ceiling instead. Meaningful calculations of reality can be made by looking at the interactions that are out of sight in the unmanifest. The totality of nature lies there, embodied in fields of virtual mass-energy. The principles of infinite correlation and all possibilities that I mentioned in relation to the intelligence of the human mind are expressed to their fullest extent in the unmanifest. All the possible universes that could exist actually do exist there, and they make up the totality of the "real" universe.

Physicists hold the unmanifest to be almost impossible to grasp intuitively. The universe has properties that our intellect cannot come to terms with outside the special language of mathematics. Speaking of this new reality, the physicist Michael Talbot remarked that it is "not only queerer than we think, but it is queerer than we *can* think." For instance, the idea that space-time came out of the unmanifest means that something exists that was there "before time began" and is "smaller than small and greater than great." These ideas seem like utter contradictions, and when we read similar things in the great Eastern traditions, we feel rather overwhelmed. However, the principles are actually quite simple to understand once your mind begins to accept the possibility of a flexible reality.

The key is to think of nature's intelligence as exactly like our intelligence. Then the new physics makes perfect sense. If I walk into a room and see a friend sitting in a chair, he might look up and say "Hello." But existing inside him are infinite numbers of things he could have said or done at that precise moment. He might have said "Albuquerque" or stood on his head. All these possibilities reside in him in unmanifest form, and they are all there at every single instant. Also, his entire unmanifest self, mind and body, is working all the time to correlate any potential thought, word, or action, even though I observe just a few of these when I interact with him. And because his DNA encodes my friend's entire development and is an encyclopedia of human evolution, we can even say that his past and future are contained in the person I see here and now.

Because the intelligence of the universe and the intelligence of the self are the same, the new physics turns out to be a great support for the main point of this part of the book, that reality can be changed once you reach the level of the self. What the new physics calls the unmanifest or virtual state of reality is what we call our selves. The universe and the human organism are united at the level of intelligence, and the source of intelligence is the self. The property that makes the universe and the self the same is called self-referral by Maharishi Mahesh Yogi. This idea expresses the most basic fact about intelligence, that intelligence operates within itself. We saw self-referral at work in "spontaneous remissions." These are cures in which an impulse of thought from the self, moving through the mind-body connection, cures the material parts of the body.

Self-referral gives a beautifully simple way to explain every act of creation. So long as we think that mind and body are separate entities, then using a thought to change the body seems impossible. But once we see that consciousness is simply working through various aspects of itself to reach other aspects of itself, then everything becomes clear. As Maharishi observes, "For all the laws of nature to be generated from their common source, that source must have the properties of infinite dynamism and self-referral; it must have the ability to create from within itself. These are the qualities of consciousness." The source of creativity is within ourselves and nowhere else. It can change reality because intelligence, our intelligence, makes reality out of itself.

This is not a surprising conclusion given what we now know of creation. Even the "hard" sciences are constantly studying feedback loops and self-regulating mechanisms. These are generally recognized as the essential mechanisms at work in preserving equilibrium in all living systems, in forming stars, galaxies, and black holes, and in creating the Big Bang itself. The hard sciences are standing on the doorstep of self-referral. Once you agree that your self is intelligent, then all creation is within your grasp through the principle of self-referral: "Curving back within myself I create again and again," as the Bhagavad Gita says.

Prescientific man in many cultures grasped this principle very well, and there is considerable evidence to show that because of this his world was much more creative and alive than the one we take for our given reality. Here is an incredibly rich description of self-referral from an ancient Indian text, the Mundaka Upanishad:

> That which cannot be seen and is beyond thought
>   which is without cause or parts,
>   which neither perceives nor acts,
>   which is unchanging, all-pervading, omnipresent,
>   subtler than the subtlest,
> That is the eternal which the wise know to be
>   the source of all.

> Just as a spider spins forth its thread,
>   and draws it in again,
> The whole creation is woven from Brahman,
>   and unto It returns.
> Just as plants are rooted in the earth,
>   all beings are supported by Brahman.
> Just as hair grows from a person's head,
>   so does everything arise from Brahman.

This passage and others like it have puzzled interpreters for generations, because they did not grasp the practical truth it contains. *Brahman* is the Sanskrit word for "great," and it means "that which is the reality of everything," in other words, intelligence. Once we understand that, this verse is absolutely clear. It is saying just what we have discovered throughout our discussion: that the only reality is infinite intelligence, creating every part of the universe effortlessly out of itself.

35

Introduction to Transcending — The Technique of Meditation

Within you there is a stillness and a sanctuary to which you can retreat at any time and be yourself.

— Hermann Hesse, *Siddhartha*

Be still and know that I am God.

— Psalm 46:10

I HAVE LAID THE GROUNDWORK for demonstrating that we can change our reality through creative intelligence. To show that this is a practical, living reality, I turn now to certain events that occurred in my life in the autumn of 1980, events that rapidly and drastically changed my world view.

Browsing through a discount bookstore in downtown Boston, I picked up a paperback on Transcendental Meditation. The author, Jack Forem, whom I subsequently came to know as a good friend, presented a means of experiencing the transcendent through a simple mental technique. The term *transcendence* had fascinated me when I read it in books, but it had always been abstract for me, since nowhere had I come across anything that said it was easy to experience. As I understood it, the realm of transcendence was the realm of "pure existence," "pure consciousness," and "pure Being." I think I am not alone in saying that such vocabulary baffled me. In many of the great Eastern traditions, these exalted terms are used, however, to apply to everyday, ordinary people:

Pure Being, thinking to itself, "May I become many, may I take form," created light. Light, thinking to itself, "May I become many, may I take form," created the waters. The waters, thinking to themselves, "May I become many, may I take form," created the earth. In this way, the whole universe was born from pure Being, that Being which is the subtlest essence of everything, the supreme reality, the self of all that exists — that thou art.

These are the words an ancient Vedic text from India puts in the mouth of a father speaking to his son when he comes of age, but as a grown man, I could only be intrigued by what they might mean. I knew from my readings in growth psychology that Abraham Maslow had called all peak experiences transcendental as well, and to a physician they sounded absolutely amazing:

There is the truest and most total kind of visual perceiving or listening or feeling. . . . It is quite characteristic in peak-experiences that the whole universe is perceived as an integrated and unified whole. . . . In my own experience, I have two subjects who, because of such an experience, were totally, immediately, and permanently cured of (in one case) chronic anxiety neurosis and (in the other case) of strong obsessional thoughts of suicide.

Maslow was understandably so impressed by such experiences that he equated them with all the revelations, illuminations, and ecstasies described by the saints of the world. Yet once again, there was no way given to have such experiences, and their descriptions made them sound like visitations, certainly not like everyday realities.

Motivated by reading this book on Transcendental Meditation, I went to the local TM center in Cambridge to hear an introductory lecture. I discovered that I needed to approach transcendence and meditation in a completely different way. Like most people in the West, I had notions about meditation that were vaguely negative to begin with. I never formulated my feelings into definite objections, but they tallied with a list drawn up by Dr. Lawrence Domash, a professional physicist and an excellent writer about Transcendental Meditation. He observed that most people assume

(1) that meditation involves concentration or controlling the mind; (2) that meditation is meant for a few select individuals with specialized lifestyles, notably the hermit, the deeply religious, and the passive mystic, all of whom are willing to withdraw from society completely; (3) that meditation is difficult and can be successfully mastered only after years of practice; and (4) that meditation "enlightens" people through some sort of self-hallucination and holds no practical benefits for ordinary life.

These views are still common in our society, and even when vaguely held they prevent many people from giving meditation a second thought. The lecturer in Cambridge, who looked reassuringly normal, made the point that not all forms of meditation are alike, and this makes immediate sense, given that several dozen cultures in the East have practiced quite different styles of meditation for thousands of years. The main points of the lecture itself were as follows: (1) the technique taught by TM is easy to learn and absolutely effortless to practice — in fact, effortlessness is the key to its success and popularity; (2) transcending is actually a process and has its origin in the mind's natural tendency to seek more charming experience; (3) becoming a meditator requires no religious belief or philosophical orientation, and no change in lifestyle other than devoting fifteen or twenty minutes to the practice, morning and evening; and (4) the primary benefits of the technique come from expanding the conscious capacity of the mind and removing deeply placed stresses from the body, both of which happen automatically, beginning with the first meditation.

I must confess that I did not entirely accept everything I was being told, but the lecturer appeared to be a very honest, intelligent person who believed completely in the technique. I decided to learn. The results from the outset were immediate and obvious to me. I realized that by learning to transcend, I was consciously opening the psychophysiological connection via a mental technique.

I was creating health.

Since then I have looked more deeply into what the process of transcending exactly is. I discovered that consciousness has become a subject of considerable scientific study since Maharishi began teaching the TM technique three decades ago. (More than three million people worldwide have learned it, including almost one million Americans, according to the TM organization.) Serious research papers have been presented and published by scientists interested in the technique, and now the compiled research runs to four volumes. Because transcending involves opening up and making use of the mind-body connection, TM promotes changes in the entire mind-body system of exactly the kind we have been discussing in this book.

Essentially, with TM the brain adopts a much more coherent style of functioning. The brain wave activity promoted by the process of transcending was not recorded before TM came to be studied. Something of the same kind, however, had been seen in just the peak moments Maslow describes when a person solves a problem, engages in creative activity, or makes a wonderful discovery. There is an overall correlation of signals from both hemispheres and all locales of the brain, and a subjective feeling of freedom, relaxation, happiness, and complete acceptance of the environment. Maharishi has pointed out that inspiration and discovery do not create this brain activity; the brain activity creates them. This is entirely in keeping with what we know about creating health: in order for intelligence to grow and bring positive changes, new channels have to be opened for it. Apparently, that is exactly what happens during meditation by transcending.

Like mind and intelligence, transcending is not a thing, it is a function. It involves the entire physiology, but specifically it works through the central nervous system. In a landmark paper from 1971 on the psychophysiology of meditation, Dr. R. Keith Wallace, then associated with the School of Medicine at the University of California, Los Angeles, described the major changes that occur in the physiology when a person transcends. During the time that the technique is being practiced, the body shows signs of deep relaxation, such as slower breathing, reduced oxygen consumption, and a decreased heart rate. The metabolic activity of the body, directly measured by how much oxygen is being used to burn fuel, dropped to levels deeper than those found in deep sleep. This was one of the most striking findings and something unique to valid transcending. Normally the body requires five or six hours of sleep to reach a point where oxygen consumption drops by around 12 percent. Meditators showed a decrease of 16 percent on the average, and the time needed was ten to twenty minutes. (Later experiments conducted with experienced meditators showed that many could drop to a level of rest twice as deep as that of sleep almost the minute they closed their eyes.)

While the body was relaxed, however, the mind remained alert. The brain waves of the meditators, measured by an EEG (electro-encephalogram), indicated a state of complete wakefulness that actually increased during the meditation session. The brain was not being highly active, however; it was lively, alert, and quiet at the same time. This led Wallace to conclude that meditation induces a "wakeful hypometabolic state," which is the physiological description of the process of transcending. The subjects themselves report feelings of alertness, inner silence, deep relaxation, and tranquillity.

All subsequent studies have corroborated the finding that these effects begin with the first meditation and become cumulative over time until the relaxed state of expanded consciousness is maintained throughout the day. It appears that transcending acts upon the central nervous system in such a way that the system becomes accustomed to being in the state of self-awareness — TM is tapping the powerful force of habit. The long-term benefits are remarkable in all areas of life. Since hundreds of studies exist — TM centers carry them in published form — and since we already know the benefits of achieving self-awareness, I will simply list some highlights:

1. Improved health, including reductions in hypertension and levels of cholesterol in the blood. Meditators qualify for the lowest available health insurance rates, and a recent report indicated that they use their insurance 50 percent less often than comparable groups.

2. Spontaneous reduction in the use of alcohol, cigarettes, and

recreational drugs. This indicates that smoking, drinking, and drug abuse fell off without any effort, simply from a lack of desire.

3. Dramatic improvements in performance on tests measuring intelligence, creativity, motor skills, and learning ability. Considering that adult IQ is considered fixed by many authorities, this result is particularly interesting as an indication of what intelligence can accomplish when stress is removed from the central nervous system. In the initial studies, college and high school students made better grades after learning the TM technique. Since then, a private school affiliated to Maharishi International University has been founded in Fairfield, Iowa, all of whose students are taught to meditate. The results are astonishing. Even though the school has an open admissions policy, its students consistently score in the ninety-ninth percentile on standardized tests in all grades. The upper school (high school) ranked first in the state of Iowa, whose school systems are consistently among the top five in the country. This shows the remarkable achievements possible when transcending is introduced to nervous systems that have not been fatigued by years of stress.

4. Reversal of the aging process. When TM was initially studied, certain indications of hormone concentrations in the blood during meditation were the reverse of those associated with aging. This was confirmed in 1982 in a pioneer study that showed that meditation seems to reverse aging. Biological aging is a complicated process, but it can be closely measured by a standardized test that looks at blood pressure, hearing ability, and near-point vision, all of which deteriorate as people age. It was found that subjects who had meditated less than five years had a biological age, on the average, that was five years lower than their actual age, while those who had meditated more than five years had a biological age twelve years lower than their actual age. This means that a person of fifty would have the physiology of a thirty-eight-year-old. Nothing in medicine can match this result, and it appears that this process improves even beyond these averages — one subject at seventy years of age had the physiology of someone in his thirties.

These are findings for groups of meditators, usually studied over a short time period. Individual meditators, whose nervous systems have become habituated to the process of transcending for long periods of time, now report many of the same experiences that Maslow discovered in the happiest, healthiest, most creative 1 percent of the population. The experiences include long durations of inner silence, joy, expanded awareness, tremendous friendliness, love, and compassion, heightened creativity, dramatically improved sensory responses, and many other signs of a consciousness that is indeed in contact with pure Being and realized self-awareness.

I am convinced that Transcendental Meditation provides an effortless technique for reaching the level of the self. From that level, the mind channels its own infinite intelligence to achieve so many benefits in all aspects of life. In essence the body clears itself of accumulated stress spontaneously, and as more channels are opened for the flow of intelligence, more of our true human potential emerges. We have already seen that a few people in every society are gifted with a physiology that can maintain health, happiness, positive emotions, and a sense of creating life as it is meant to be lived. But every physiology wants to do the same thing. Transcending activates the pathways that ill health, stress, wrong habits, negative attitudes, and defective experiences have caused to deteriorate. (There is even some preliminary research showing that intelligence may be enhanced at the level of the DNA itself.) Through transcending, the rest of us can live up to the best of us.

36

Spontaneous Right Action
and Higher States of Consciousness

> Our normal waking consciousness, rational conscious-
> ness as we call it, is but one special type of conscious-
> ness, whilst all about it, parted from it by the filmiest of
> screens, there lie potential forms of consciousness en-
> tirely different. We may go through life without sus-
> pecting their existence; but apply the requisite stimulus,
> and at a touch they are there in all their completeness.
>
> — William James

WHAT YOU WANT and enjoy should also happen to be good for
you. This concept, which has cropped up several times in our discussion, gives the only effortless criterion for evaluating our
thoughts and desires. We know that we want to promote in ourselves only what is positive, progressive, evolutionary, and life enhancing. The intention to live according to that standard has not
yet transformed itself into a reality, however; it cannot unless the
psychophysiological connection is in the habit of spontaneously
rejecting all wrong styles of functioning and promoting only right
ones. Since every single thought, as we have seen, corresponds to a
distinct organization of every part of the physiology, how can we
possibly control the billions of unseen neural connections, cell
functions, hormone and enzyme interactions, and so on that go
into every single thought we have? Obviously we cannot. The intellect cannot control what it is not even aware of.

Yet we must achieve "spontaneous right action" — the phrase
comes from Maharishi Mahesh Yogi — if we expect to achieve

perfect health and self-fulfillment. How do we judge whether an action is right or wrong in the first place? We look at the results. Every thought carries at its inception a means of attainment. As the thought unfolds itself into speech or action, it either turns out right or it falls short of what we wanted. If one channel of spontaneous right action has been cultivated, we have what we call a skill. A surgeon does not put in some stitches and then take out the wrong ones; his hands have the skill for doing the right thing every time. The same is true of concert pianists, who do not after all get to smile and take back their wrong notes. We are all used to spontaneous right action of this sort — we all have skills. The psychophysiological connection is coordinating our thoughts and actions all the time.

Therefore, if we want to progress in spontaneous right action, we only need to cultivate and perfect what the mind-body connection is already doing naturally. The process of shaping reality is natural to us; it is the basic function of the share of infinite intelligence that we know how to use. We can conceive of knowing how to use more of this intelligence, so much more that our own reality would be progressive, evolutionary, and life enhancing. That would be a perfected state of spontaneous right action. It is also the only valid, practical meaning for "higher states of consciousness." To be able to create consciously a positive reality all the time is to be in a higher state of consciousness.

We have arrived at quite a marvelous conclusion, for it becomes obvious that we do not have to do anything different to achieve higher states of consciousness from what we are doing every day. Our intelligence is shaping reality every day; we only have to do it better.

If we look closely at our actions, we discover that judging an action by its results is not really effective in determining whether it was right or wrong. Consciously eating the "right" diet does not ensure that you will not be struck by illness; it only lowers your risk. Also, our actions are complexly interwoven with each other and deeply embedded in a complex human environment. The conscious mind cannot possibly judge whether every word we say promotes peace, compassion, well-being, and harmony. Life is far too complex for that, and it would impose a great strain on our lives if we had to pause and judge everything we did. (That is why schools of positive thinking and self-observation create unnatural strains on the awareness.)

Words and actions cannot be taken back. Therefore, even if we did have the ability to know immediately that an action was wrong, what good would it do us? What is done is done. Clearly the only way to act and speak correctly is to have the skill for it. Thoughts, words, and actions have to be right at their inception. If they are right at the outset, at the level of the self, then nature will automatically direct the necessary functions closer to the surface. When a pianist wants to play Mozart, he simply sits down and plays. His intention, coupled with the skill he has cultivated in his physiology, spontaneously creates the desired results.

Now we see with full clarity why the "self" has been so important in creating health. Intentions for achieving health, happiness, love, or any other aspect of reality must start somewhere. We become aware of them as thoughts, but that is not where they start. People differ in whether they have clear thoughts or fuzzy thoughts, deep or shallow thoughts, refined or gross thoughts. Yet everyone who possesses intelligence creates reality. It is a process of intelligence; therefore, it must begin where intelligence begins, and that is at the level of the self. The self is simply the most general level of intelligence. If we want our desires to become living realities, they must be life-supporting at the level of the self.

Do we need to improve the self? No — the self is by definition our most general level of intelligence. Since intelligence is already infinite and capable of running the entire universe, how can it be improved? What needs to be improved — this has become obvious by now — is the psychophysiological connection to the self. Intelligence is absolutely flexible, yet absolutely rigid at the same time. If you set up one channel for it, it follows that channel by habit until you redirect it, which is something we have discussed in detail already. But setting up one habit after another is highly inefficient. Using the principle of the highest first that I introduced in chapter 34, we should be able simply to contact the level of the self and then let intelligence do the rest of the work for us.

Apparently that is exactly what happens in the process of transcending. When scientists hear that meditators have achieved the remarkable benefits I mentioned in the last chapter, they are at a loss to find a reason for it. You do not seem to be doing anything when you transcend. Yet you are doing something. The Upanishads contain a famous passage: "Know that, knowing which, all else is known." This is what transcending accomplishes. It channels the awareness to the self, allows the self to be known, and then nature does the rest.

Your brain and central nervous system are already coordinating billions of physiological functions every second with incredible efficiency. Given the optimal initial conditions, they will tend to work much better automatically. Your deepest beliefs, operating at the level of collective consciousness, completely control the reality you accept through your senses. Given the optimal initial conditions, they too will produce a more coherent, intelligent, and evolutionary reality automatically. This explains in our modern language what the great traditions of wisdom have been communicating since humanity came to consciousness: know your self, and all of nature will be yours.

Let us consider the process of transcending more closely. The physiological description for it is "a hypometabolic wakeful state." This means that the body is rested while the mind is alert. Physiologists who have studied meditation in great detail tend to accept the claim that transcending deserves to be called a separate state of consciousness. During the process of meditation, the functioning of the central nervous system is not the same as it is in waking, dreaming, or sleeping, and the differences become dramatically pronounced when advanced meditators are studied. Their breathing while they meditate is much shallower than it is in a waking state, their brain waves display overall coherence unique to transcending, and the carbon dioxide levels in their blood are patterned quite differently from what physiologists have previously measured. This validates what the ancient Vedic texts in India tell us when they say that the self is beyond waking, sleeping, and dreaming.

But what does "beyond" mean? One of the greatest and most common misconceptions about the process of transcending is that it takes you out of reality. Sometimes the phrase "transcending the self" is used, but it is quite incorrect. The process of transcending brings you *closer* to the self. What you are getting away from are your random thoughts and habitual stress responses. The injunction of the sages to "leave the self and arrive at the Self" does not mean that we leave our personalities somewhere down the road. The self is our intelligence. Exchanging the "self" for the "Self" means to convert our small share of intelligence into an infinite share. Genius, for example, is greater selfhood. When Maslow describes the "godlike" feelings that come over people during peak experiences, he is observing the total change of awareness that occurs when a small intelligence suddenly realizes that it is capable of infinite expansion.

The process of transcending thoughts is quite mechanical. In the Transcendental Meditation technique a specialized, meaningless sound, or mantra, is used to allow the awareness to reach subtler levels of thinking. The vehicle of using a sound happens to be quite efficient. The awareness dips into subtler and subtler levels until all thought is transcended, or gone beyond. At that point, the awareness has reached, to use Maharishi's phraseology, pure awareness or pure consciousness, the level of the self. To put it another way, at every level of thought there is a corresponding state of the psychophysiological connection. Each one is like a plateau at which specific organizations of thoughts, neural connections, hormone responses, and so on are operating.

When the awareness transcends and perceives itself as reaching a subtler level of thinking, what is happening physically is a new projection of mind-body functioning. The thought is only the tip of the iceberg; the vaster reality consists of billions of coordinated physiological processes. When the awareness eventually reaches the state of silence or pure consciousness, the mind-body connection is projecting its optimal state of functioning — nothing is random or stressful. In fact, in this state, stresses can be released from the central nervous system because there is no longer any physiological tendency to promote them. At this level of the self, the physiology automatically heads in the direction of optimal functioning because that is the tendency of the flow of intelligence by its very nature.

Consciousness is the total projection, in other words, of the activity in your nervous system. Each projection is a distinct thing, just as each thought is distinct. What are called "higher states of consciousness" must also be distinct levels of brain functioning; otherwise, they could not be stabilized. They would have no physiological reality. In fact, everything that happens during the process of transcending must have a physiological correlate or it would not be real. The mind would simply be fooling itself. When we say that awareness is expanded or that intelligence has found a new channel to flow through, something real has to be happening.

I should mention here that the TM technique is obviously not the only way to transcend. The process is as old as human consciousness and has been occurring spontaneously to a few gifted people throughout history; that is why Maslow could connect his recent studies of peak experiences to transcendental experiences of the past. The TM technique is efficient, easy, systematic, and works for everyone. It has been thoroughly documented at every stage by science and requires no nonsecular orientation. For these reasons, I strongly recommend it. If I had discovered anything comparable while researching this book, I would be recommending it.

Beyond Transcending:
Higher States of Consciousness

Each state of consciousness creates a new reality. Each one is a plateau of mind-body functioning; each one brings a different aspect of infinite intelligence into play. Thanks to the endless flexibility of the central nervous system, our intelligence can suppress parts of itself and bring other parts into play as it wants to. When you are asleep, your intelligence activates the biochemistry of sleep. When you are awake, it activates a different biochemistry. There is no limit to the possibilities, yet at any one moment not all of them are apparent. The absent ones are not unreal, they are just out of sight. The great American psychologist William James, speaking of other states of consciousness, wrote that "at a touch they are there in all their completeness."

We see exactly this when transcending becomes an ingrained habit. Transcending ushers in new states of consciousness that carry completely different realities with them, as different as waking, dreaming, and sleeping. These are the three states of consciousness. Transcendental consciousness, which is reached through meditation, we could call a fourth state. It is the silent state of self-awareness in which brain activity is fully coherent and effortlessly coordinated with the body to produce the flow of pure intelligence. Therefore, it is the same for everyone, generally speaking, just as sleep is the same for everyone and dreaming is the same for everyone. Of course we all have different kinds of dreams and no two dreams are alike, so we would expect the same variation when people experience transcending. No two experiences of it are exactly alike, yet the general outlines are the same so far as the psychophysiological connection is concerned.

When transcending has been systematically cultivated over a period of time (which varies widely from person to person), the awareness retains its contact with the self throughout the other three states of consciousness. When the brain waves of a meditator are measured on an EEG, the coherence that was characteristic of transcending is seen to be maintained even during waking, dreaming, and sleeping. This is how transcending is able to bring its benefits; it persists in the physiology of the central nervous system even after the twenty minutes of meditation are over. In other words, intelligence prefers it. The attention recognizes this preference as a feeling of clarity, openness, inner tranquillity, heightened vitality, and mental silence maintained with activity.

In the terminology of Transcendental Meditation, which is in keeping with a long tradition, this new state is called cosmic consciousness. The word *cosmic* here means total or all-around, signifying that transcendence has been totally infused. It is the state in which for the first time the infinite flow of universal intelligence has been activated. Transcending cleared the stage; in cosmic consciousness the full drama of life begins.

The physiologist can actually confirm that cosmic consciousness is distinctly itself and qualifies as a fifth state of consciousness. Not only is brain wave coherence maintained around the clock, as I mentioned, but other biological changes appear. The amount of the amino acid phenylalanine increases in the blood, and the amount of such stress hormones as cortisol from the adrenal glands decreases. There are a host of correlated changes from pituitary hormones, including thyroid-stimulating hormone, growth hormone, and prolactin. As more people are verified as being in a state of cosmic consciousness, researchers hope that new substances might appear that the stressed physiology was suppressing; this seems a real possibility. It would extend the psychophysiological connection to higher states of consciousness.

With cosmic consciousness, our search for the self has ended. When this state is reached, the person can create his own reality. The channels of infinite intelligence are completely coordinated and nature is ready to act. Whatever thoughts of compassion, love, hope, and self-fulfillment that may arise are translated into everyday life. Life becomes completely positive and harmonious. The depths of consciousness, with all their vitality and creativity, come to the surface of life. All action is spontaneous right action. Every desire directs itself to the highest goals of life; therefore, following the principle of the highest first, one has only to have a desire and nature does all the work. To be in cosmic consciousness is to create life from one's complete intelligence.

We need to be clear that this is a necessity. Our good intentions and positive emotions have done nothing to stabilize a wholly positive reality. At the level of collective consciousness, we have all agreed to fear, hatred, war, sickness, suffering, and death. They have become our inherited reality, and every day we spend the inheritance. Change is only possible at the level of the self, as we have abundantly proved in our discussion. If life is to be set on a higher plane, we must find that plane. It exists in our minds and in our physiology. It is the possibility for cosmic consciousness.

Nothing is more important for humanity today than for everyone to understand that he can easily reach this state. We are all creating reality already. With a slight shift of emphasis, effortlessly brought on through the process of transcending, we can create a reality that deserves to be called human. Our everyday, normal actions are not yet right; witness the prevalence of the silent killers, heart disease and cancer. People who develop these conditions have not consciously decided to harm themselves. They have adopted the normal lifestyles that everyone around them participates in. Yet many of their daily actions amount to sheer self-destruction. Their awareness has not comprehended this. No one feels that he himself is responsible for disease, much less human suffering and war. Everyone simply acts from his own level of awareness; this is true of every person, regardless of how right or wrong, good or bad, we think his actions are.

In fact, it is totally irrelevant what we judge our own actions to be. We simply act as our level of consciousness dictates. If we want to change our existence meaningfully, then we must change our level of consciousness. We *must*. Talking, thinking, arguing, hoping, and praying for a better life only satisfy a superficial level of the mind, and hardly that. When real change occurs, it is real; it is not a mood. It has nothing to do with keeping watch over your problems or trying your best to control your impulses. They are your reality. Indeed, desires are the way to cosmic consciousness.

Desire is the father of reality. What you desire is simply what you want to do. Desires are the impulses of intelligence rising into your consciousness, and therefore they are all you have to go on. You are led from moment to moment by desires. So we come back to the essential point: what you want and enjoy should also happen to be good for you. And this can only be a certainty in cosmic consciousness.

The process of coordinating the mind and body to the utmost degree can be hastened. By learning to transcend, the nervous system has reached a state where thinking becomes much more successful. The impulses of thought can rise directly to the level of action. In this way, a desire becomes instantly realized. In fact, all enlightened thoughts arise in this efficient, unhindered way; no friction is encountered in the form of stress or contrary impulses. Such perfected thoughts are called *sidhis* in Sanskrit, and it is possible to practice their mechanics even before the mind is in an enlightened state.

The *sidhis* make it possible actually to do something in the transcendent, to move around in it. I have found it tremendously useful to cultivate this refinement of the process of transcending (for several years I have been following the program of TM-Sidhis, which is a natural adjunct to the Transcendental Meditation technique), but since learning to transcend is absolutely necessary in order for these perfected thoughts to have any meaning, I will save them for later writings. To show how far mind-body coordination can be extended, however, let me mention that *sidhis* are applied to expand the positive emotions, such as love and compassion; to refine greatly all the senses, allowing direct appreciation of nature at the finest levels; to acquire further metabolic relaxation through control of the breath and other body functions; and to draw on nature for support in all endeavors. They are the technology of the future for anyone who has mastered transcending.

After Enlightenment

Just as transcending is the prerequisite for gaining cosmic consciousness, cosmic consciousness is the prerequisite for attaining all higher evolution. The higher states of consciousness take off from here. I will not spend a great deal of time discussing them, but they are the supreme levels of human experience. Those who achieve them are the guides of humanity and the progenitors of everything we think of as noble and dignified in humanity. When we have made the shift in our consciousness that turns sickness, suffering, violence, and death into bad dreams, into nonrealities that do not deserve the name human, then the higher states of man's life will become natural. They are the spring of our year, but we are still in winter.

Once a physiology has stabilized cosmic consciousness, it is said to be enlightened. In a literal sense, there are no more dark corners. The various stresses and malfunctions that allow intelligence to misfunction and create disease have been removed. Where once there was darkness, now there is light, which is simply intelligence. At our best moments of love, health, happiness, and creativity, we are already enlightened. Having those moments extend into every day's reality is cosmic consciousness. We do not have to acquire any new abilities to become enlightened; we only have to allow nature to clear the way for the mind-body connection to operate at optimal efficiency.

Maharishi Mahesh Yogi has given us some beautiful descriptions of the higher plateaus of normal human existence. In the sixth state of consciousness, one level above cosmic consciousness, "we gain the ability to perceive the finest relative [values] on the surface of every object while maintaining unbounded awareness." This is called refined cosmic consciousness. In cosmic consciousness the awareness has made the breakthrough, but once it has time to become refined, everything that the senses can see, touch, hear, smell, and taste becomes supremely beautiful. In the seventh state of consciousness, "every object is perceived in its infinite value and the gulf between the knower and the object of knowing is bridged. Knowledge is complete and full." Maharishi terms this unity consciousness and remarks, "There is no further development beyond this unified state because the perceiver and the object of perception have both risen to the same infinite value." In unity, the wholeness of life begins to be lived and enjoyed as a daily reality.

A great deal of harm has been done to life by our not knowing that these possibilities exist. Now that we know, it would do more harm to continue as if the old reality, with its continual threats, were permanent. The old reality is not permanent. It is shifting at the level of collective consciousness and giving way to something altogether new and better. We will examine the evidence for that in the closing chapter, which is a vision of oneness.

37

One Is All, and All Is One

Every grain of sap contains the full value of the whole tree.

— Maharishi Mahesh Yogi

To see a World in a Grain of Sand
And a Heaven in a Wild Flower,
Hold Infinity in the palm of your hand
And Eternity in an hour.

— William Blake

REALITY EXISTS because you agree to it. Whenever reality shifts, the agreement has been changed. In the history of science this has been called a paradigm shift. This idea was first proposed by the noted historian of science Thomas Kuhn in his book *The Structure of Scientific Revolutions,* where he described a paradigm as a scientific framework that explains reality. It is like a fence that encloses all the scientific facts of the moment; it embodies the current world view. Up until 1453, for example, everyone agreed that the sun rose in the east and set in the west. This view was attested to by the senses, and all the events that needed to be explained by science fitted in accord with this fact. In the fifteenth century, however, a shift took place. Observers began to take notice of new happenings in nature. Since nature is infinite and always present, it would be truer to say instead that men began to notice things that they had overlooked or had been unwilling to perceive. When Copernicus hypothesized that the sun did not move through the sky but that the earth moved around the sun instead, a revolution took place — the old paradigm was overthrown.

Revolution is the right word for this process, because everything that the old reality explained had to be reinterpreted. Once the apple cart turns over, everything in it has to be picked up again. The point for us to see is that no one thought he *wanted* the paradigm to shift. With perfect hindsight we see that the theories of Copernicus, Galileo, and Newton brought about an incredibly interesting and rich reality. People at the time did not think so, and everyone who had a stake in orthodox opinion, all the right-thinking, serious people heartily opposed the "new science."

The paradigm is not a fact in itself, but a concept. In order for reality to shift, the concept must be accepted, and that can only happen at the level of collective consciousness. Geniuses on the order of Newton and Einstein lead the way — one could say that they precipitate the new reality first — but everyone needs to follow if the shift is to be accepted as "really" happening. In our own day, more than half a century after the General Theory of Relativity was first proposed, its insights are not common knowledge. Until fifteen years ago relativity was thought far too difficult for high school students to understand, and many physics teachers themselves have only a dim grasp of it. Yet it is reality. Reality is what we agree upon, and anyone who has looked at nature through the eyes of Einstein and the next two generations of new physicists understands that a great shift has occurred whose ramifications will eventually topple every outpost of received opinion.

Nature is infinite, and therefore no scientific paradigm can explain all of it. Once you shift your view of reality, nature has a lot more of reality to show you. We must fully understand that reality can change whenever our view of nature and her infinite possibilities decides that a change should be made. Most people do not consider this. They think, for example, that it is *true* that the earth goes around the sun and not vice versa.

In fact, this question is sheerly a matter of perspective. Both the earth and the sun are suspended in empty space. Their motions are caught up in the larger rotational motion of our galaxy, and the galaxy itself is rushing away from the source of the Big Bang at tremendous speed.

Whether you believe that the earth moves around the sun or that the sun moves around the earth depends upon where you stand, what you want to know, and how you go about knowing it. Medieval astrologers were primarily interested in matters that could be understood very well by placing the earth at the center of their astrological charts. However, if you want to be entirely precise, it is better and simpler to devise a solar system in which the sun is at the center, because then all the planets move around it in simple, regular ellipses. Under the old system, the planets had to back up and undergo "retrograde motion," as the term went. To the eye looking at the night sky, that is exactly what the planets seem to be doing. That was their reality, and so it stands on astrological charts to this day.

People will not accept facts that do not fit into their world view. If they are told or if they even see for themselves that cancer can be spontaneously cured, that portions of the brain can be removed without loss to the mind, that a mentally retarded man can sit down and play a Tchaikovsky piano concerto without ever taking lessons, that congenital idiots can perform intricate mathematical calculations in an instant, or that human beings can walk on burning coals (just to pick a few newsworthy items you may have read about in the last two years), these events still have no reality until something more basic happens. The more basic things needed are, first, a new explanation that works better than the old explanation, and second, a shift in collective consciousness to create fully the new reality.

I have been proposing here that perfect health is a reality for anyone, that everyone can expand his share of infinite intelligence. Whatever the mind of man can conceive, the mind of man can accomplish. An enormous range of nature not explained by the current world view and the current science is about to unfold itself. As it does, the collective consciousness will discover a human reality far richer than what it knew before. That is in fact the only reason for humanity as a collection of individual minds to change its view of reality; the possibility for growth is inherent in us. Our minds are part and parcel of nature, and so we share in the force of evolution that causes everything in nature to progress, to unfold more and more of the possibilities of intelligence.

It is understandable when any new paradigm meets with resistance. Every paradigm explains everything. Our present paradigm, which states that it is "impossible" for the inner reality of a person and the outer reality of the world to harmonize fully, is now accepted as correct. The new paradigm will also explain everything, but it will explain *more*. Here are some signs of the shift and the things that are coming to be explained:

1. When a number of laboratory rats are trained to accomplish a new task, such as learning to run through a complicated maze, some researchers have found that rats in other parts of the world are able to carry out the same task more easily. These other rats are not related to the first batch genetically; they are all simply rats. They have no physical connection or communication with the original batch. They seem to learn more quickly just because the first batch already learned the task.

2. Even more fascinating is the story of some Japanese monkeys that live wild on the island of Koshima off the Japanese mainland islands. This scientific tale has become rather famous because of Lyall Watson, an English biologist who reported the incident in his book *Lifetide*. (He has written a series of books, all of them spellbinding, on the events in nature that challenge thinking at the frontier of science.)

Just after World War II, Japanese scientists studying these monkey tribes left food on the beach in the form of sweet potatoes, which the monkeys relished. However, the monkeys found it difficult to eat the sweet potatoes because of the sand that covered them after they were dropped by the scientists. Then, in 1952, a certain young female monkey, named Imo by the scientists, hit upon the idea of taking the potatoes down to a stream and washing them. The intelligence it took to find such an original solution to the problem Watson calls genius, comparable to man's discovering the wheel. The other young monkeys watched Imo, caught on to her trick, and soon many were washing their potatoes, too.

In time, all the juvenile monkeys were washing their dirty food, though interestingly adult monkeys over five years of age only did so if they were directly imitating a younger monkey. In the fall of that year a large number of monkeys on Koshima were washing their food, but now in the sea, because the "genius" of the tribe, Imo, had discovered that salt water not only washed the food but gave it a flavor the monkeys liked. Watson arbitrarily sets the large number of monkeys doing this at ninety-nine. Then one evening, the hundredth monkey learned to wash his food. Watson reports a remarkable phenomenon that resulted:

> But the addition of the hundredth monkey apparently carried the number across some sort of threshold, pushing it through a kind of critical mass, because by that evening almost everyone in the colony was doing it. Not only that, but the habit seems to have jumped natural barriers and to have appeared spontaneously, like glycerine crystals in sealed laboratory jars, in colonies on other islands and on the mainland in a troop at Takasakiyama.

According to the theory of evolution proposed by Darwin and held in modern form by geneticists, this is an impossible event. How can a trait be passed on spontaneously in the same generation of a species, much less all at once and at several places separated in space? The glycerine in jars Watson mentions is an example of the same kind where the new behavior was not even learned by a living species. It is extremely difficult to cause glycerine to turn into crystals, yet after the first successful achievement of inducing crystallization, glycerine spontaneously crystallized in sealed jars in other laboratories. As in "the hundredth monkey phenomenon," intelligence was acting in a self-referral manner, leaping across barriers in an "impossible" way. But this is simply the natural behavior of intelligence — it affects itself by itself and through itself. It knows no absolute barriers. Intelligence of course does not just leap out of bounds. It respects its own pathways. However, it knows how to set up new pathways as well. New realities are created when the need for them arises.

Watson's most telling comment was, considering what we have discussed about collective consciousness, "It may be that when enough of us hold something to be true, it becomes true for everyone." Einstein said much the same thing about his ideas on relativity theory.

3. If collective consciousness is real, then you should be able to do something with it. In this light, the Transcendental Meditation organization has conducted experiments to see whether collective consciousness can be stimulated and made more life supporting. The results of the experiments are fascinating, since they give evidence for the new paradigm that is quite factual. Dozens of these experiments have been conducted so far. I will just report the highlights.

A 1976 study published by Dr. Candace Borland, a psychologist, discovered that when 1 percent of a city's population has started to meditate, the crime rate in that city spontaneously begins to decline. Using a group of eleven American cities in which 1 percent were documented as having learned the TM technique, Dr. Borland found decreases in crime of as much as 16 percent in one year compared to comparable cities where, as in the rest of America at the time, the crime rate was rising. This study has been replicated many times over using hundreds of towns and cities, always with similar results.

In 1979 a large group of TM meditators gathered at the University of Massachusetts at Amherst for an assembly that included periods of group meditation every day. Physiologists at Maharishi International University in Iowa measured the brain activity of subjects who were meditating in Iowa at the same time. Without having any contact with the Amherst group or any knowledge about when the Amherst group performed their meditation (an advanced meditational technique, the TM-Sidhis, was involved), the Iowa meditators showed increased brain wave coherence exactly at the time when the Amherst group began practicing its techniques. The coherence was not present either before or after this specific period.

In the winter of 1983 a very large group of meditators, numbering around seventy-five hundred, assembled in Iowa for another conference that included group practice of TM and the advanced TM-Sidhis technique. Sociologists studied more than a dozen variables that might be influenced at the level of collective consciousness. Using extremely reliable and sophisticated statistical techniques, they found that remarkable changes occurred. During just this period, the stock market reversed itself after months of stagnation and began to rally, moving upward in almost a straight line until the last day of the conference. As soon as the group meditations of the seventy-five hundred ended, the market immediately fell and took almost a straight-line decline. Although not so dramatically, other indices changed as well: automobile accidents declined during the period, hospital admissions declined, crime rates decreased, and signs of international conflict were reported less often in news reports.

These results seem impossible unless one understands that reality is shaped at the level of collective consciousness, in which case these results are fascinating and highly promising for making human reality positive and progressive. Over the last fifteen years similar results have been verified in dozens of experiments, testing the effects of meditation on the national crime rate, military conflicts, automobile accidents, incidence of disease, and various measures of general quality of life. According to the current paradigm, these are completely unrelated variables. There is no reason why they should improve together, nor is there any reason why they should improve spontaneously in correlation to the meditation of groups of people far away.

The reason such results are possible is that intelligence is one. If the individual intelligence can spontaneously cure a disease process, bring more peaceful and loving thoughts, remove internal stress, and point the mind toward positive attitudes, then there is nothing to stop this process from happening on a larger scale. All reality is shared, and what is reality for one is reality for all. At the level of collective consciousness, we have agreed to this one reality. We have to, for it is only through shared intelligence that any reality can be created at all — intelligence is one thing, only expressing itself in infinitely different channels.

* * *

The new paradigm is coming together from many diverse sources. We have already touched upon the new physics, which began the paradigm shift through the theory of relativity. Some advanced thinkers in physics now propose that collective consciousness is the only hypothesis that can explain the universe we see and accept as real. A British biologist, Dr. Rupert Sheldrake, is pioneering the study of the "hidden force" that might account for such things as the hundredth monkey phenomenon. He proposes that changes in the forms of plants and animals can in fact be caused at a subtler level than that of DNA. In other words, rather than relying only on the physical make-up of the genes, he is looking at their abstract quality, the information that they encode. As we have discussed, the genes are not simply physical; they transmit the collected knowledge of all evolution. Dr. Sheldrake has proposed that there exist fields of information that actually form life into the shapes we see. These "morphogenetic fields" shape life before the physical shape manifests itself. In essence, they are nature's version of thoughts.

The idea of a field underlies much of the thinking in the new physics. What were once seen as separate electrons or separate light waves are now seen as manifestations of infinite fields. The fields are the "real" reality; what we see are just local events popping up out of them. Sheldrake is extending the field concept to biology, and TM researchers are taking it into the realm of human consciousness. That is the way the paradigm spreads, moving from one area to another until all the apples from the spilled apple cart have been picked up again.

Why should consciousness be a field? The TM scientists Drs. R. Keith Wallace, Michael Dillbeck, and David Orme-Johnson proposed the idea of a consciousness field in order to explain just the experimental results mentioned here. How can two brains respond to each other at a distance? How can meditation by a small or large group of people cause crime rates to drop? Armed with hundreds of reliable factual findings and needing to explain them, the TM scientists have taken advantage of the new paradigm. If we think of human consciousness as an infinite field that each person is one local expression of, then it becomes plausible that one part of the field can affect another part. That is exactly how fields work. A compass anywhere in the earth's magnetic field will align itself with that field spontaneously — it will point north. So if the process of transcending allows individual minds to settle down and reach a state of maximum brain coherence, it seems logical that other human minds might feel the effect. A "hidden force" in the field of consciousness is shaping the effects that then pop up as reality. The force is not a mystery once we understand that it is awareness. Awareness, channeling intelligence at the level of the self, brings the benefits of meditation. On a larger scale, it brings about benefits to the expression of intelligence that is society.

The TM researchers have given a name to the general effect that they are studying, calling it the Maharishi effect. Maharishi Mahesh Yogi, in his teachings about consciousness, was the first to predict that the transcending process could cause changes over a distance, which is the prime characteristic of a field effect. He had also speculated that only a small number of people would be necessary to produce the effect. The basis for that speculation came from physics again, where instances were well known in which only a small number of particles have to change in order for the whole to change. For example, if you magnetize about 1 percent of the atoms in a bar of iron, the rest of the bar will become magnetized. The same is true in chemical reactions; as soon as a small percentage of a solution has reacted, the rest of the reaction follows almost instantly. Many other physical effects, including the laser, work in the same way.

The same logic was then extended to human consciousness. Lyall Watson had speculated that if enough of us think something is true, it becomes true for all of us. The Maharishi effect apparently shows that it does not take many of us. The significant breakthrough came with the discovery that the effect must take place on a deeper level than that of thought. During the process of transcending, a meditator is not thinking of crime, war, disease, and so on, trying to conquer them. He is simply exposing his awareness to the level of the self, to consciousness as it exists before thoughts come into being. Having done that, intelligence spontaneously does the rest. The TM researchers comment that "this remarkable new technology for creating coherence in collective consciousness could potentially lead not only to the improvement of the quality of life in cities, as the crime studies cited above suggest, but also to the resolution of international conflicts and the establishment of world peace."

In other words, the effect can spread. One quiet, peaceful, coherent consciousness has tremendous power — so the lives of Gandhi, Mother Theresa, and many who are not famous show. If our consciousness can grow to match theirs, then the same influence will spread farther. If we can deepen our awareness beyond even what they experience, then the influence will last.

Lasting healing and lasting peace are real only at the level of our being. So long as what we are is isolated from nature, we will not be helped by nature, and that includes our own nature. The great German philosopher Martin Heidegger has said that the threat that hangs over humanity comes from within. It comes because man wills himself against the flow of nature, or Being, when he is meant to live with it: "Human nature resides in the relation of Being to man." This Being is our source. Attempting to live outside it disrupts everything: "The world becomes without healing, unholy."

People fear the danger of the nuclear bomb, but this danger, of a world without healing, is *the* danger, Heidegger declares. All of the other threats — war, disease, hatred, death — have come from it. This is where a new world view brings the end of all threats. "But," Heidegger says, "where there is danger, there grows also what saves." We have only to point ourselves back to our source, back to our being, and nature will heal itself.

We do not have to be scientists to understand why a new reality is pushing its way through our minds. A world without healing is intolerable to us. Illness is not natural. It is not only that we suffer from it. At the deepest core of ourselves, illness offends us, because it limits our freedom, and the one thing that intelligence can never tolerate the loss of is freedom. The heart expands at the possibility of health, happiness, and love. When we begin to create health, the unholy world erected by our minds transforms itself into a higher reality, the world of the heart. The human heart contains all beings through its compassion. It is the world's inner realm, greater than all of objective space. Our thoughts are like a counselor who whispers into the ear of a king. However wise he is, he is not the king. The king is heart and mind, emotion and intelligence, all in one. Because every person alive contains these within himself, every person can rule himself. At the level of our being, we have all the power we could possibly need to create a new reality.

Once we welcome our awareness back to its source, the problems of living disappear. The realization comes that the problems do not in fact exist. Out of that realization, a different world arises. It is healed and it is holy.

Epilogue: The Future

·

NEW REALITIES ultimately are not that new. The concepts presented in this book are only one aspect of a whole "science of life" that goes back thousands of years in human awareness. It is not limited in time or place, but there is a living tradition centered on it in India known as Ayurveda. The name comes from two Sanskrit roots, *ayus* or "life," and *veda,* or "knowledge." I have related its few basic premises already: (a) Nature is intelligent, (b) man is a part of nature, and therefore (c) the same intelligence permeates both. Taking these few ideas as self-evident facts, Ayurveda unfolds a wealth of technologies to maintain health, not simply in man, but in all the aspects of nature that share its infinite intelligence.

Ayurveda uses its techniques in the service of balance. When nature is unbalanced, the whole is endangered by disruptions in its parts. To be healthy, all natural beings must interact with nature through open and balanced channels of intelligence. The value of change, or dynamism, must be balanced with nonchange, or stability. Our word for this is *homeostasis* — the balance of functions that keep a living organism's physiology in equilibrium. The knowledge of homeostasis that modern medicine has gained in the last half-century is fully compatible with Ayurveda. Only, a bridge has to be built from one world view to another.

In a general way, that has been the purpose of this book. Ayurveda has volumes to say about the relationship of food, behavior, biological rhythms, environment, and thought, all of which it examines in relation to the whole. And because man and nature are completely compatible in the Ayurvedic system, the physician who understands Ayurveda can command a vast array of herbs, purifying therapies, and rejuvenation techniques to alleviate disease and promote longevity in the most natural way possible. When correctly practiced, Ayurveda has no side effects. It operates from the level of intelligence that is common to man and nature. Indeed, Ayurveda sees man as nothing less than the embodiment of every power in nature, and fully as infinite. One famous aphorism from the Ayurvedic texts declares that "Ayurveda is for immortality." Human potential is carried to the ultimate.

The elegant, simple, and effortless techniques of Ayurveda will occupy my writing in the future. I want to say here that they all begin in consciousness; therefore, by describing the process of transcending, I have already told you of the most powerful therapy known to the science of life. The last part of this book has placed its focus on consciousness as a field. Because it cannot be separated from the universal field that gives rise to reality, our consciousness field contains all possibilities. The future, insofar as I can see into it, will unfold this truth. It holds the master key to perfect health and happiness. It is at the core of shaping a new reality.

More specifically, I see our shared reality unfolding along these lines:

1. More and more people will gain access to an understanding of the field of consciousness.

2. Because of a rise in consciousness, we will witness a steady

decline in the number of deaths from today's common diseases —
cancer, stroke, hypertension, heart disease — and fewer fatalities
from accidents of all kinds.

3. People will live longer and healthier lives. Alcohol, cigarettes,
and recreational drugs will loosen their hold on people's lives. Science will advance aided by subjective realization of man's true
nature. Spontaneous right action will become commonplace as a
normal trait.

4. Groups of people who have learned the process of transcending will activate the field of consciousness more and more deeply,
and with more and more benefit to themselves. Highly developed
individuals will emerge who actually experience and understand
self-awareness. Peak experiences will no longer be accidental.
These highly developed people will be creating health to the optimal extent — they will maintain the peak.

5. As the dynamics of group consciousness are further explored,
they will be applied successfully to solve social problems on the
widest possible scale. Crime and social deviance will dramatically
decrease. Prosperity and progress will be dramatically advanced.
World peace will become a practical possibility and not just a
hope. What the mind of man conceives, it will find the power to
accomplish.

Every tradition of wisdom holds that our scope is unlimited.
The field of human life is a field of infinite possibilities. Inside
every man is a god in embryo. It has only one desire. It wants to
be born.

Acknowledgments

I would like to thank all those who took this book along the road to publication: John Halberstadt, who was so helpful with the first steps; Carla Linton, who showed faith all along the way and never faltered in her dedication; and Ruth Hapgood, my editor at Houghton Mifflin, whose humor, skill, and tact made the final stages of publication so effortless.

Very special thanks go to my wife, Rita, and my children, Mallika and Gautama, whose love is my energy.

As this book was going to press, I received valuable assistance from Huntley Dent. His deep friendship, refined criticism, and literary skill continue to guide my every project.